ORAL LEUKOPLAKIA

DEVELOPMENTS IN ONCOLOGY

Volume 8

Previously published in this series:

1. Cleton F. J. and Simons J. W. I. M (eds): Genetic Origins of Tumor Cells. 1980. ISBN 90-247-2272-1
2. Aisner J. and Chang P. (eds): Cancer Treatment Research. 1980. ISBN 90-247-2358-2
3. Ongerboer de Visser B. W., Bosch D. A. and van Woerkom-Eykenboom W. M. H. (eds): Neuro-Oncology: Clinical and Experimental Aspects. 1980. ISBN 90-247-2421-X
4. Hellmann K., Hilgard P., Eccles S. (eds): Metastasis: Clinical and Experimental Aspects. 1980. ISBN 90-247-2424-4
5. Seigler H. F. (ed): Clinical Management of Melanoma. 1982. ISBN 90-247-2584-4
6. Correa P. (ed): Epidemiology of Cancer of the Digestive Tract. 1982. ISBN 90-247-2601-8
7. Liotta L. A. and Hart I. R. (eds): Tumor Invasion and Metastasis. 1982. ISBN 90-247-2611-5

ORAL LEUKOPLAKIA

Jolán Bánóczy

Clinic of Maxillo-Facial Surgery and Dentistry
Semmelweis University Medical School
Budapest, Hungary

1982

Martinus Nijhoff Publishers

The Hague · Boston · London

Translated by I. Koch

English translation edited by M. B. Edwards

The distribution of this book is handled by the following team of publishers:

for the United States and Canada

Kluwer Boston, Inc.
190 Old Derby Street
Hingham, MA 02043
USA

for all other countries

Kluwer Academic Publishers
Group Distribution Center
P.O. Box 322
3300 AH Dordrecht
The Netherlands

for Hungary, Albania, Bulgaria, China, Cuba, Czechoslovakia, German Democratic Republic, Democratic People's Republic of Korea, Mongolia, Poland, Roumania, Soviet Union, Democratic Republic of Vietnam, and Yugoslavia

Kultura, Hungarian Foreign
Trading Co., H-1389
Budapest 62,
P.O. Box 149
Hungary

Library of Congress Cataloging in Publication Data

Bánóczy, Jolán.
Oral leukoplakia.

(Developments in oncology; v. 8)
Includes index.
1. Leukoplakia, Oral. I. Title. II. Series.
[DNLM: 1. Leukoplakia, Oral. W1 DE998N v. 8/
WU 280 B2190]
RC815.B34 616.3'1 82-3467
ISBN-13: 978-94-009-7566-8 AACR2

ISBN-13: 978-94-009-7566-8 e-ISBN-13: 978-94-009-7564-4
DOI: 10.1007/978-94-009-7564-4

Joint edition published by

MARTINUS NIJHOFF PUBLISHERS
P.O.B. 566, 2501 CN the Hague, The Netherlands
and
AKADÉMIAI KIADÓ
1054 Alkotmány u. 21, Budapest, Hungary

CONTENTS

This monograph is dedicated to Dr. L. Sugár, my tutor in scientific research, in grateful appreciation of the selfless support received from him in my studies of precancerosis which I had the privilege to start as his assistant.

I also owe a tribute to the memory of the late Professor K. Balogh, my beloved first master, who opened my eyes to the pleasures of scientific work and gave me invaluable help and advice for two decades.

The Author

PREFACE

Clinical and pathological observations have unequivocally indicated an increase in the incidence of malignant neoplasia during the last two decades. Despite important advances in surgery, radiotherapy and chemotherapy, mortality from tumours still tends to increase. Cancer research has therefore concentrated not only on early diagnosis and therapy but also, in line with recent trends in medical science, on the prevention of oncogenesis. One efficient prophylactic approach is the treatment of preblastomatoses, which include the preneoplastic lesions of the mouth. The most frequent oral precancerosis, leukoplakia, has been studied extensively during the last 20 years with regard to its pathogenesis, clinical course, and response to therapy.

In Hungary, studies of oral leukoplakia have a century-long tradition. The term leukoplakia was coined by the Hungarian dermatologist Ernő Schwimmer who recognized the precancerous nature of the condition and its relationship to tobacco smoking exactly 100 years ago. In the middle of this century another Hungarian scientist, Károly Balogh established that most leukoplakias have two stages, — reversible and irreversible — and that early lesions may heal spontaneously after the elimination of irritational factors. The incidence of leukoplakia in random population groups was determined for the first time in the world by the Hungarian investigator Pál Bruszt, and reported to be 3.6%. Subsequent studies in other countries confirmed a range of 0.2–8.1%, depending on geographical and environmental conditions, way of life, and relevant habits.

The definition of leukoplakia has been much disputed because white patches of the oral mucosa may arise in many different pathological states. The conflicting opinions have been reconciled by the W. H. O. Collaborating Centre for Oral Precancerous Lesions (of which Jolán Bánóczy is a member), through the definition of leukoplakia as a white patch on the oral mucosa which cannot be classified as any other entity. It should be noted that the original term leukoplakia has been internationally accepted and used without synonymous substitution in any language.

Various aspects of leukoplakia such as frequency and clinical features have often been studied in samples collected from single examinations made at one given time. However, certain aspects, especially the rate and etiology of malignant transformation, can be covered more satisfactorily by longitudinal studies based on annual or bi-annual examination of the patients over long periods. Such studies enable the clinical course to be followed, and results of treatment to be evaluated. Follow-up studies of this kind were initiated in the Clinic of Maxillo-Facial Surgery and Dentistry, Dental Faculty of Semmelweis University Medical School, Budapest by Jolán Bánóczy and myself. In this collaborative study we established the rate of malignant transformation, and the significance of the site of the lesion. Bánóczy made an independent contribution of important information on various aspects of oral leukoplakia from long-term studies of a very large group of patients. She presented evidence of the transformation of one clinical type into another, assessed the frequency of regressive and progressive changes, and showed that malignant transformation was closely related to the type of keratinization, since cancer most frequently developed from parakeratinized lesions. She also described the ultrastructural characteristics of oral leukoplakia with special reference to clinical type and histological structure.

Benign hyperkeratosis of inflammatory origin often cannot be differentiated from early carcinoma in situ by clinical features alone. Closer investigations into the nature of precanceroses are therefore imperative, and it is expected that the information which will emerge from such studies will contribute to a better knowledge of carcinogenesis, and thereby to more efficient therapy and prevention of neoplastic diseases.

László Sugár

INTRODUCTION

THE DEFINITION, NATURE AND FREQUENCY OF ORAL LEUKOPLAKIA. OBJECTIVES

Leukoplakia has long been recognized as the most frequent precancerous lesion of the mouth. The term "leukoplakia", originally proposed by the Hungarian dermatologist Ernő Schwimmer in 1877, has been the subject of recurrent dispute. This is because its literal meaning is "white patch" (Gr. leukos = white; plakia = patch) which describes a clinical entity. Yet lesions so designated may have many different histological forms. In view of this, some authors have attempted to define leukoplakia in histological terms (Kollar et al. 1954, Fasske et al. 1958, Hansen 1959, Thoma and Goldman 1960, Waldron and Shafer 1960, Shafer and Waldron 1961, Hellinger et al. 1963, Morgenroth 1963, 1964). Kramer (1969, 1976) and Cooke (1975) have applied the term exclusively to white patches with histological evidence of epithelial dysplasia. The histological definition of leukoplakia is, however, complicated by the fact that not all lesions satisfying the histological criteria for leukoplakia will appear clinically as a white patch (Shafer 1967). The dispute concerning the definition of leukoplakia is enduring. In 1963 Sprage found that 36 % of American oral pathologists used leukoplakia as a clinical term and 40 % as a histological one.

To reconcile conflicting opinions, the W.H.O. Collaborating Centre for Oral Precancerous Lesions proposed in 1978 that *the term leukoplakia should be used to describe a clinical entity, that is a white patch of the oral mucosa which is not removed by tubbing and not classifiable as any other oral disease* (e.g. oral lichen planus, leukoedema, candidiasis, white sponge naevus and morsicatio buccarum et labiorum), while microscopically leukoplakic lesions should be described in internationally approved term. This definition has been generally accepted by contemporary investigators in both clinical stomatology and oral pathology (Pindborg 1971), and I have relied upon it in this monograph. Mention should be made of recent attempts (Hornstein 1977*a*, *b*) to integrate this definition into the dermatological (nosological–etiological) classification of leukoplakia, which was elaborated in part by Greither (1970). In that scheme, the current definition of leukoplakia would fit the category designated as "exogenous irritative leukoplakia".

Table 1

Epidemiological observations on the incidence of leukoplakia

Author(s)	Year	Country	No. of persons examined	Type of community	Prevalence (%)
Gerry et al.	1952	Guatemala	2,004	rural	0.4
Mehta et al.	1961	India	4,734	urban	3.5
Balogh and Huszár	1962	Hungary	103	rural gipsies	40.7
Bruszt	1962	Hungary	5,613	rural	3.6
Kovács	1962	Hungary	500	urban	2.0
Atkinson et al.	1964	New Guinea	3,996	rural	8.1
Pindborg et al.	1965–66	India	30,000	urban	1.6–3.3
Zachariah et al.	1966	India	10,000	urban	2.4
Pindborg et al.	1968	New Guinea	1,226	rural	4.6
Bánóczy et al.	1969	Hungary	16,332	rural	0.57
Wahi and Mital	1970	India	7,286	rural	5.2
Mehta et al.	1969	India	50,915	rural	0.2–4.9
Gangadharan and Paymaster	1971	India	203,249	urban	0.7
Sonkodi and Tóth	1973	Hungary	1,071	urban	1.21
Axell	1975	Sweden	8,696	urban	3.2
Silverman et al.	1976	India	57,518	urban	11.7
Wilsch et al.	1978	GFR	4,000	urban	2.2

Data from the world literature on the prevalence of leukoplakia are shown in Table 1. The first reported screening of random population groups was undertaken in Hungary by Bruszt in 1962. Of the inhabitants of seven villages over 14 years of age, a total of 5,613 persons, 3.6% had leukoplakia and 0.14% a benign oral tumour. Bánóczy and her collaborators (1969) launched a stomato-oncological screening programme within the framework of compulsory pulmonary screening amongst 16,332 persons in two villages. Of these, 0.1% had a benign oral tumour and 0.57% had leukoplakia. Sonkodi and Tóth (1973) found oral leukoplakia in 1.21% of 1,071 textile mill workers, examined in a screening study. It follows that in Hungary the prevalence of leukoplakia has ranged between 0.57 and 3.6% in random population groups. This approximates to the prevalence found in other countries.

Oral leukoplakia satisfies the definition of a precancerosis as formulated by Cabanne (cit. Kuffer 1972) at the Fourth Congress on Cervico-Facial Carcinoma (Lyon 1971): "... precancerosis is understood as a condition which, although free from any indication of an infiltrating carcinoma, is significantly more liable to cancer development than the similar intact tissues, as judged from clinical and pathological observations", while the W.H.O definition says that a precancerous lesion is considered "as a morphologically altered tissue in which cancer is more likely to occur than in its apparently normal counterpart" (Pindborg 1980). The precancerous nature of oral leukoplakia has been substantiated by scores of studies but the precise factors responsible for malignant transformation, which only occurs in a small proportion (5–7%) of leukoplakia, are still not fully understood, neither has the group of definitively precancerous leukoplakias been described precisely. It therefore seemed worthwhile to study the following aspects of oral leukoplakia in a large group of patients:

1. Clinical features, rate of malignant transformation, and factors promoting transformation.
2. Cytological and histological features, and their relationship with clinical type.
3. Segregation of strictly precancerous lesions by the identification of changes from one clinical type to another, by analysis of cases with histological evidence of epithelial dysplasia and by ultrastructural studies.
4. Differential diagnosis from other white lesions of the oral mucosa.
5. Therapeutic approaches and their efficiency.

The patients studied were from the Clinics of Maxillo-Facial Surgery and Dentistry and of Conservative Dentistry, Semmelweis University Medical School Budapest. From a total of 979 subjects, included in our clinical follow-up study, 520 had oral leukoplakia, 326 had lichen oris, 70 had glossitis migrans, 45 had white sponge naevus and 18 had lesions attributed to cheek biting. In many cases, lesions were examined by cytological, histological, electron microscopic and morphometric (stereological) methods.

The clinical, cytological and histological studies primarily served diagnostic and therapeutic purposes, while the electron microscopic and morphometric examinations served as an experimental approach to aspects that remain to be clarified by research.

At the first examination each patient was interviewed to obtain a case history with special reference to possible etiological factors, such as the type of smoking habit and quantity of tobacco smoked, alcohol consumption and syphilis. In addition to the case history, we recorded the patient's oral condition at admission, and also the presence of any mechanical irritating factors in the mouth. The electrical potential difference was measured in each case that had metal restorations and/or fillings (Inovay and Bánóczy 1960*a*,*b*, 1961), and differences exceeding 50 mV were regarded as significant. Each lesion was photographed, and occasionally stomatoscopic examinations were performed. Cytological smears were taken in each case, and detection of fungi was attempted in smears and/or by culture if there was a clinical suspicion of candidiasis. Histological examination was performed if (*a*) there was clinical suspicion of malignancy at the first examination, or (*b*) the lesion failed to heal within 2–3 months at the latest after the elimination of irritating factors and/or the application of conservative treatment (irreversible leukoplakia; Balogh 1956). The patient was sent for haematological examination if there was a clinical suspicion of anaemia or some other disease of the haemopoietic system.

The records kept of each patient included the results of all investigations, treatments and observations made at follow-up examinations at intervals of 1–2 years. The same principles of examination and recording were employed in the cases of oral lichen planus, leukoedema exfoliativum mucosae oris (white sponge naevus) and morsicatio buccarum et labiorum (cheek biting).

The information that emerged from these long-term studies is presented in this monograph in a logical sequence as followed by the clinician handling a case. Thus the first chapter deals with the results of longitudinal studies, with special regard to observations concerning the precancerous nature of oral leukoplakia. This is followed by a detailed description of possible etiological factors, and of the clinical examinations which presuppose some knowledge of these. Complementary microscopic (histological and cytological) examinations are subject of a further chapter, after which there follows a description of ultrastructural (transmission and scanning electron microscopic and morphometric) studies which are in the orbit of fundamental research. Concerning the differential diagnosis of leukoplakia from other white lesions of the mouth, detailed descriptions are given of those well-known to us from longitudinal studies on large groups of patients. Last but not least, separate chapter is devoted to description of my experiences and those of my co-workers in the treatment of leukoplakia, in the hope that other investigators engaged in this problematical task may profit from it.

Although this monograph is far being a complete review of the topic, I hope that this contents, based on diagnostic, therapeutic, and research experience of large groups of patients, can contribute to better knowledge of factors that promote the malignant transformation of oral leukoplakia, and thereby to the prevention of oral cancer. This has been the primary motive of all my related work over a quarter of a century.

CHAPTER I

RESULTS OF CLINICAL FOLLOW-UP STUDIES IN ORAL LEUKOPLAKIA

Longitudinal studies of the rate of malignant change in oral leukoplakia were first reported in 1957 (Sugár and Bánóczy 1957). Since then similar studies have been carried out in several other countries (Table 2). To summarize the results, the frequency of carcinomatous change in oral leukoplakia has been found to vary between 1.4 and 6% over observation periods of 3 to 25 years. Of a total of 2,112 patients in these studies 96 (4.5%) developed malignant lesions.

The results of my follow-up studies on oral leukoplakia since 1957 have been described in several reports (L. Sugár and Bánóczy 1957, 1959, 1969, Bánóczy and L. Sugár 1968*b*, 1972, Bánóczy 1977). The last report (Bánóczy 1977) was based on the clinical study of 670 patients but, as detailed examinations with additional methods were not possible in that particular group, the observations described in this monograph apply to the 520 patients available for study in 1972 (Bánóczy and L. Sugár 1972). As the clinical

Table 2

Frequency of cancer development from oral leukoplakia in different countries

Author(s)	Country and year	Period of observation (years)	No. of patients with leukoplakia	Percentage of malignant transformation
Sugár L. and Bánóczy	Hungary, 1957	11	86	5.8
Skach et al.	Czechoslovakia, 1960	6	71	1.4
Mela and Mongini	Italy, 1966	11	141	3.5
Einhorn and Wersäll	Sweden, 1967	20	782	4.0
Pindborg et al.	Denmark, 1968	9	248	4.4
Silverman and Rozen	U.S.A., 1968	5	117	6.0
Sugár L. and Bánóczy	Hungary, 1969	22	324	5.5
Roed-Petersen	Denmark, 1971	12	331	3.6
Bánóczy and Sugár L.	Hungary, 1972	25	520	5.9
Pindborg et al.	India, 1975	7	170	3.5
Bánóczy	Hungary, 1977	30	670	6.6

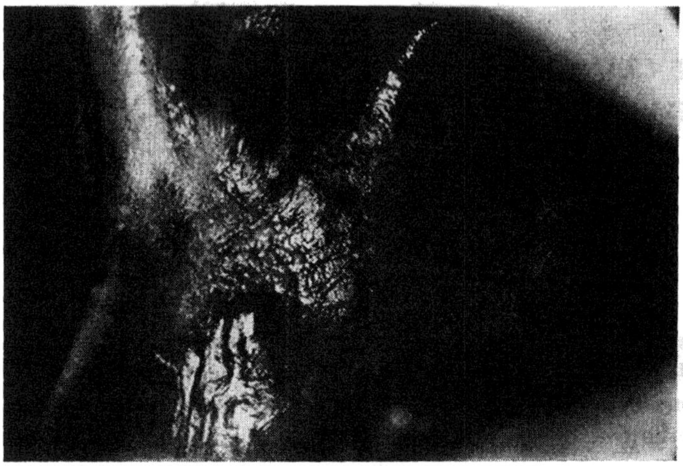

Fig. 1. Simple leukoplakia in the commissure of a 40-year-old female patient. Within the characteristically triangular lesion the mucous membrane is lustreless, white, and thick

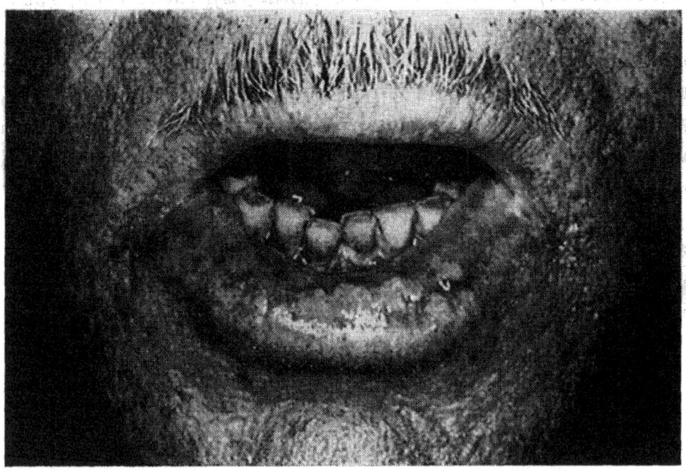

Fig. 2. Simple leukoplakia developed from cheilitis actinica on the lower lip of a 72-year-old farmer

findings were similar in the two periods, the conclusions drawn from the use of supplementary methods of examination can be regarded as generally relevant.

From a total of 722 patients with oral leukoplakia seen in the Clinic of Maxillo-Facial Surgery and Dentistry of the Semmelweis University

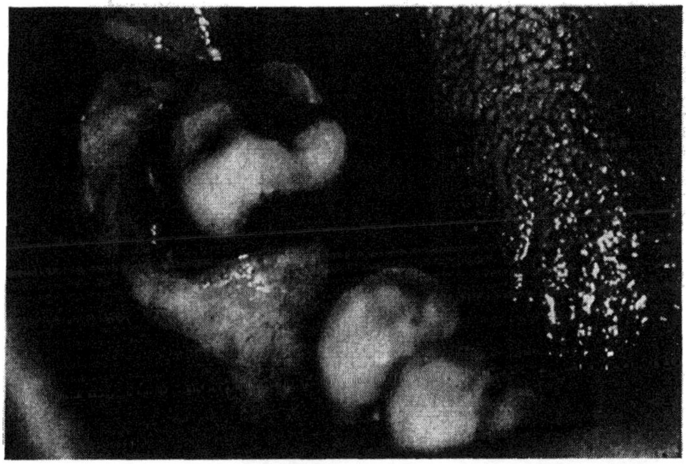

Fig. 3. Simple leukoplakia. The 55-year-old male patient, a heavy smoker, developed the hyperkeratotic lesion on the alveolar mucosa, at the site of a missing lower molar

Medical School, Budapest, over a 25-year period 520 (72%) were available for follow-up examination. Of the 202 patients not available for follow-up, 41 (5.8%) died of some other disease and 161 (22.2%) did not present for re-examination; some of these had left the country.

The periods of observation were from 1 to 25 years, with a mean of 8.7 years. The clinical methods of examination are described in the introductory chapter of this volume.

Various authors have proposed schemes for the classification of the clinical types of oral leukoplakia (Prinz 1928, Hobaek 1947, Ward 1953, Fasske et al. 1958, Hahn et al. 1961, Pindborg et al. 1963, Knychalska-Karwan 1965c, Venkei and J. Sugár 1965). We have used the three-type classification elaborated by L. Sugár and myself in previous studies (L. Sugár and Bánóczy 1957, 1959, Bánóczy and L. Sugár, 1968). The following types are considered in this scheme:

Type I: *Leukoplakia simplex* — keratinized mucosa: — flat, or very slightly elevated white lesions, with a pavement- or mosaic-like hyperkeratotic pattern (Figs 1, 2, 3 and 5 as well as colour photos 1 and 2).

Type II: *Leukoplakia verrucosa* — verrucous proliferations raised above the mucosal surface (Figs 4–6 and colour photo 3).

Type III: *Leukoplakia erosiva* — erosions and fissures in a white, hyperkeratotic area (colour photo 4).

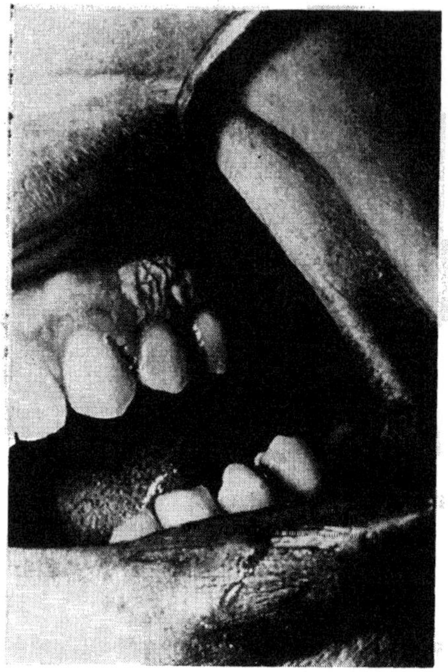

Fig. 4. Verrucous leukoplakia near to the upper premolar teeth on the attached gingiva of a 66-year-old non-smoking woman. An electric potential difference exceeding 50 mV was demonstrated between fillings made of different metal alloys

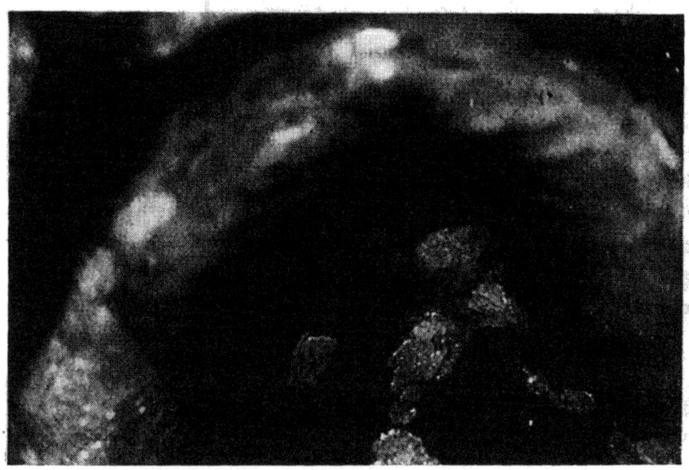

Fig. 5. Circumscribed simple plus verrucous leukoplakia on the hard palate of a 53-year-old woman who used a poorly fitting prosthesis

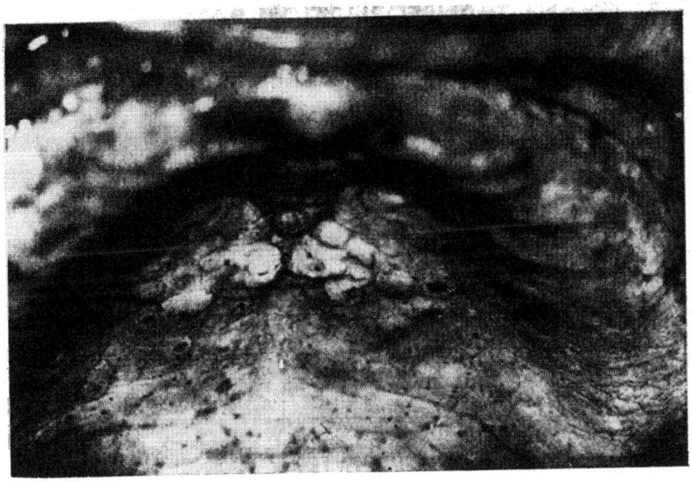

Fig. 6. Nicotinic leukokeratosis of the palate in an 84-year-old man who had smoked 8–10 pipes daily for many decades, but who did not wear a prosthesis

This scheme correlates well with the widely accepted classification proposed by Pindborg et al. (1963), in that the type termed as "homogeneous" by them includes our simplex and verrucous forms, while their "speckled" type corresponds with the form described by us as erosive (Hornstein 1977*a*).

The main purpose of our longitudinal studies was to identify the factors correlated with malignant transformation in oral leukoplakia. We investigated

— the malignant transformation rate in oral leukoplakia,
— the age and sex distribution of patients with leukoplakia and with carcinoma arising in leukoplakia,
— the site of leukoplakia and carcinoma,
— the interrelationship between the clinical type and malignant transformation, and
— the latency period.

The role of etiological factors, and the methods of treatment are described in another chapter.

MALIGNANT TRANSFORMATION RATE

This was assessed in relation to clinical state (recovered, improved, unchanged, spread) and histological evidence of cancer. Table 3 shows that among the 520 patients included in the follow-up study 176 recovered, 131 showed improvement, 135 showed no change of state and 47 showed spread of the lesion. *Carcinoma developed in 31 cases (5.9%).*

Table 3

Results of the follow-up study of leukoplakia

Result	Cases	
	No.	%
Recovered	176	33.8
Improved	131	25.3
Unchanged	135	26.0
Spread of lesion	47	9.0
Carcinoma	31	5.9
Totals	520	100.0

AGE AND SEX DISTRIBUTION

This was recorded at the first examination of patients with oral leukoplakia, and at the time of the diagnosis of carcinoma (Table 4).

The prevalence of leukoplakia tended to increase in both sexes after the age of 40 years, and to reach a peak between 50 and 59 years. Malignant trans-

Table 4

Age and sex distribution of patients with leukoplakia and carcinoma

Age groups (years)	Leukoplakia			Carcinoma		
	Men	Women	Total	Men	Women	Total
20–29	11	4	15	—	—	—
30–39	44	14	58	3	1	4
40–49	74	24	98	4	—	4
50–59	123	35	158	3	3	6
60–69	101	29	130	9	3	12
above 70	42	19	61	3	2	5
Totals	395	125	520	22	9	31

formation of leukoplakia occurred between 30 and 39 years at the earliest and had its peak between 60 and 69 years. However, the absolute numbers of patients with carcinoma within the various age groups were not completely indicative of the age-dependence of malignant change, for the age groups differed in size and sex distribution. We therefore determined from the census returns for 1960 and 1970 (Statistical Yearbook – Statisztikai Évkönyv 1960, 1970) the average size of the various age groups at the national level without consideration of sex distribution, and we calculated the numbers of patients likely to occur within each group if the condition was independent of age. The quotient obtained by dividing the actual number of patients with their computed number served as an index figure which indicated the frequency of leukoplakia in any given age group, regardless of its size. The actual and computed numbers of patients, and the quotients are shown in Table 5.

It was established that, in relation to the age distribution of the total population, *the incidence of oral leukoplakia was highest between 50 and 68 years of age in both sexes* and tended to decrease slightly after 70 years of age. The age distribution of malignant transformation could not be assessed on this basis because of the relatively low number of carcinomas.

The group of patients with leukoplakia comprised 395 men (75.9%) and 125 women (24.1%), i.e. *the sex ratio was 3 : 1.* Of the patients with malignant transformation 21 were men and nine were women, giving a sex ratio of 2.4:1. This suggests a slightly higher rate of malignant transformation among the women [9 in 125 (7.2%) against 22 in 395 (5.5%)], but the difference is not statistically significant ($0.6 < p > 0.3$).

Table 5

Computed and actual age group distribution of patients with leukoplakia (men + women)

Age groups (years) \ Leukoplakia	Computed number of patients	Actual number of patients	Quotient of actual and computed numbers
20–29	109.24	15	0.14
30–39	108.13	58	0.54
40–49	98.52	98	0.99
50–59	86.98	158	1.82
60–69	70.38	130	1.85
above 70	46.75	61	1.30
Totals	520.00	520	–

SITE OF LEUKOPLAKIA AND CARCINOMA

The site of the lesions was determined according to Roed-Petersen and Renstrup's (1969) topographical classification (Figs 7 and 8) used also by the W.H.O (1980). The lesion was regarded as commissural, if it extended posteriorly from the labial commissure over a distance of about 2 cm, usually in a triangular shape, and as buccal, if it was located in the central zone of the buccal mucosa, in the molar region and along the occlusal line.

At first examination 62.8 % of the patients had a lesion either at the commissures, or on the buccal mucosa, and 8.5 % each had lesion on the tongue or hard palate. 130 patients had lesions in several sites, usually symmetrically in the commissure and buccal mucosa.

The distribution of patients according to the site of leukoplakia is shown in falling sequence in Table 6.

Comparison of the site distribution between the sexes indicated that in men the most common site was the commissure (42 %) and next the buccal

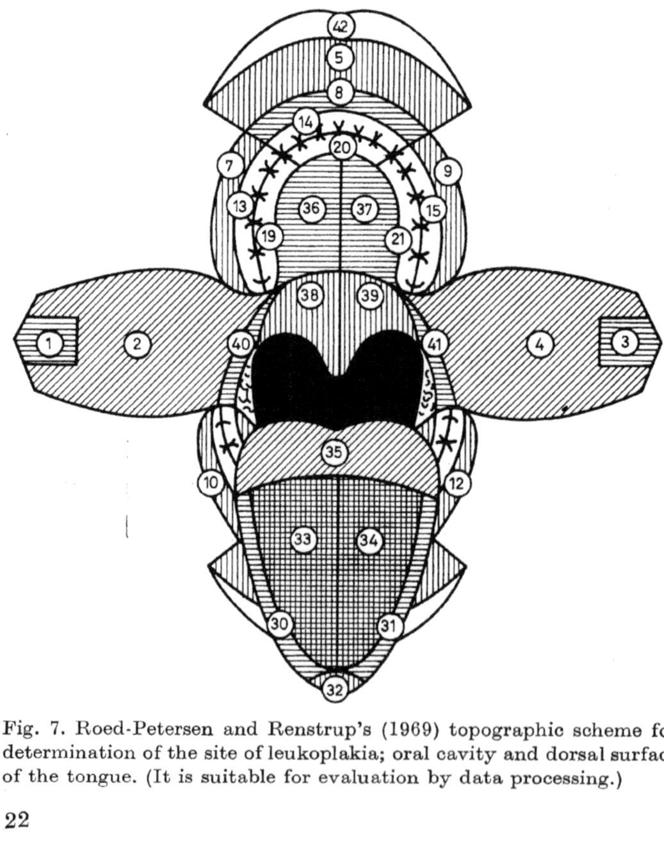

Fig. 7. Roed-Petersen and Renstrup's (1969) topographic scheme for determination of the site of leukoplakia; oral cavity and dorsal surface of the tongue. (It is suitable for evaluation by data processing.)

Table 6

Distribution of patients according to the location of oral leukoplakia

Location	Men		Women		Total	
	No.	%	No.	%	No.	%
Commissures	166	42.0	24	19.2	190	36.5
Buccal mucosa	87	22.0	50	40.0	137	26.3
Lip	28	7.1	6	4.8	34	6.5
Tongue	27	6.8	17	13.6	44	8.5
Hard palate	32	8.1	12	9.6	44	8.5
Soft palate	5	1.2	2	1.6	7	1.3
Floor of the mouth	22	5.7	8	6.4	30	5.8
Alveolar ridge	28	7.1	6	4.8	34	6.6
Totals	395	100.0	125	100.0	520	100.0

mucosa (22 %), while in women this distribution was reversed (buccal mucosa 40 %, commissure 19.2 %). The lip was more frequently affected in men (7.1 %) than in women (4.7 %), while the tongue was nearly twice as frequently affected in women (13.6 %) than in men (6.8 %).

The site distribution of carcinoma (Table 7) shows that *malignant transformation occurred most frequently [12 of 31 cases (38.8 %)] in lingual lesions,* with the cancer being located at the margin or root of the tongue. Cancer incidence was significantly greater on the tongue than in other site of leukoplakia ($p < 0.001$). Cancer developing from leukoplakia of the lip was

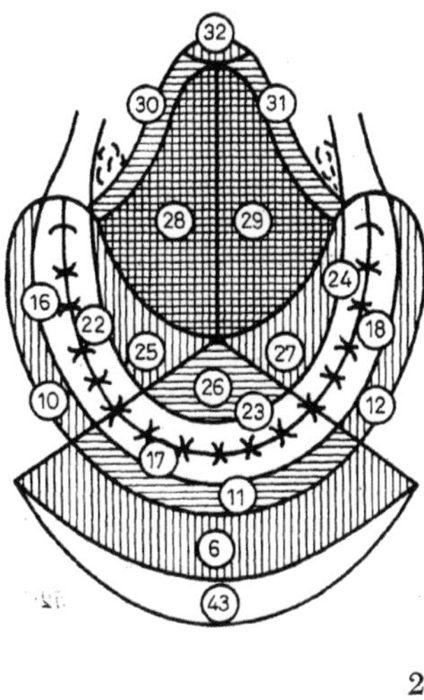

Fig. 8. The same scheme as in Fig. 7., showing the ventral surface of the tongue, floor of the mouth and the lower lip. (Also this is suitable for evaluation by data processing.)

Table 7

Distribution of patients according to the location of carcinoma

Location	Men		Women		Total	
	No.	%	No.	%	No.	%
Commissures	3	13.6	—	—	3	9.7
Buccal mucosa	3	13.6	—	—	3	9.7
Lip	5	22.7	—	—	5	16.1
Tongue	4	18.2	8	88.8	12	38.8
Hard palate	1	4.6	1	11.2	2	6.4
Soft palate	1	4.6	—	—	1	3.2
Floor of the mouth	3	13.6	—	—	3	9.7
Alveolar ridge	2	9.1	—	—	2	6.4
Totals	22	100.0	9	100.0	31	100.0

next most frequent (16.1%), while the occurrence of malignancy was roughly equal between the other sites, such as buccal mucosa, commissures, palate, floor of mouth and alveolar ridge.

Analysis of the sex distribution of cancer developing in the different sites showed that 88.8% of malignancies in women developed from leukoplakia of the tongue.

CORRELATION BETWEEN THE CLINICAL TYPE AND MALIGNANT TRANSFORMATION OF ORAL LEUKOPLAKIA

The distribution of malignant transformation in the various clinical types of leukoplakia is shown in Table 8.

Table 8

The distribution of clinical types of oral leukoplakia and role of malignant transformation

Clinical types of leukoplakia	No. of cases	Carcinoma	
		case	%
Simple	265	—	—
Verrucous	173	8	4.6
Erosive	82	23	28.0
Totals	520	31	5.9

No cancer developed in the 265 cases of leukoplakia simplex. Eight of the 173 verrucous leukoplakias (4.6%), and *23 of the 82 erosive leukoplakias (28%) underwent malignant transformation.* Statistical analysis revealed a very significant correlation ($p < 0.001$) between clinical type and malignant change. In percentage terms, 74 and 26% of the 31 carcinomas arose from erosive and verrucous leukoplakia, respectively.

LATENCY PERIOD

Latency is the time interval between the clinical manifestation of leukoplakia and the diagnostic identification of carcinoma. It is often difficult to determine the time of onset of leukoplakia, for patients do not usually notice the change. Not infrequently the lesion is recognized by the dentist. In such cases the examiner has no choice but to rely on the patients history. In the group studied by us, the latency period varied between 1 and 29 years. Latency periods longer than 10 years were relatively frequent (12 cases), indicating the importance of the time factor in cancer development (Table 9).

In this group of patients with leukoplakia, the prevalence of malignant transformation was similar to that found previously (L. Sugár and Bánóczy 1957, 1959, 1969, Bánóczy and L. Sugár 1968*b*, 1972). Other authors have given the prevalence of malignant transformation as from 1.4–6%. The 5.9% prevalence found by us therefore reaches the upper limit established in longitudinal studies. The prevalence of malignant transformation may be influenced by several factors, such as the number of the patients studied, the length of the observation period, and even by geographical factors, to judge from the dissimilar prevalences of oral leukoplakia and oral carcinoma in different

Table 9

Latency periods of cancer developing in oral leukoplakia

Years	Men	Women	Totals
>1 year – < 5 years	6	2	8
>5 years – <10 years	4	3	7
>10 years – <15 years	4	1	5
>15 years – <20 years	2	1	3
>20 years	2	2	4
Unknown	4	—	4
Totals	22	9	31

countries or continents. In Hungary, the prevalence of oral leukoplakia varies between 0.6 and 3.6 % in the different regions (Bánóczy et al. 1969, Sonkodi and Tóth 1973, Bruszt 1962*a*, *b*); in India (Mehta et al. 1969*b*) it varies between 0.2 and 4.9 %. The occurrence of oral carcinoma in Europe ranges between 1 and 5 % (Pindborg 1965), being 1.5, 2, 3 and 4 % in Denmark, Switzerland, Italy and France, respectively, and as high as 5 % of the total cancer prevalence in Hungary. This can be regarded as one possible explanation of the high rate of malignant transformation found in our follow-up studies.

Analysis of age distribution showed that the prevalence of oral leukoplakia was highest between 50 and 69 years of age, while that of carcinoma had its peak in the 60 to 69-year-old age group. This shift emphasizes the importance of the latency period and indicates that malignant transformation often takes place after oral leukoplakia has been longstanding (frequently longer than 10 years). This observation correlates well with the findings of Burkhardt and Seifert (1977). Pindborg (1978) established that women usually develop oral leukoplakia at a somewhat older age than men.

The apparently greater risk in women of malignant change in oral leukoplakia has also been observed by other authors (Gangadharan and Paymaster 1971). Roed-Petersen (1971) reported the incidence of malignant transformation as 5.8 % among women and 2.1 % in men, i.e. an even greater sex difference than the one found by us (7. and 5.5 %).

The site distribution of leukoplakia and carcinoma is very varied. The predominant sites of the former are the commissures and the buccal mucosa, but only 1.8 % of all malignant transformation (six cases among 327 leukoplakias) arose in these sites. Gangadharan and Paymaster (1971) reported similar observations. Against this, while only 6.5 and 8.5 % of leukoplakias developed on the lip and tongue, respectively, 16.1 and 38.8 % of carcinomatous changes occurred exactly in these sites. It follows that 14.7 % (five cases in 34) of labial leukoplakias and 27.2 % (12 cases in 44) of lingual leukoplakias, were subject to malignant transformation, which corresponds well with Shafer's data (1980), who found a higher incidence of carcinoma in situ in these sites.

The high frequency of cancer development from leukoplakia of the tongue (38.8 %) is relevant to an investigation by Roed-Petersen (1971), who found that 44.4 % of oral carcinomas were located on the margin of the tongue. In Hungary (Vándor 1969, 1978) 10 % of oral neoplasms were identified as buccal carcinoma, and 20–30 % as carcinoma of the tongue proper. This percentage of lingual lesions is similar to our findings.

Two-thirds of the patients with lingual carcinoma were women, thus the sex ratio was 1:2 in this particular group as against 2.4:1 for all oral carcinomas. This ratio is even higher than that observed by Ash (1962) who, in the

United States, found a higher prevalence of lingual than oral carcinoma among women too, to judge from the respective sex ratios of 2:1 and 4:1. However, our findings do not equate with the statistics of another Hungarian investigator (Vándor 1969), who gave the male/female ratio for lingual carcinoma as 5:1. The reason for this dissimilarity may be related to variation in cancer prevalence in different zones of the tongue. The apparently greater risk in women of malignant change in leukoplakia suggests the involvement of endogenous factors (anaemia, hormonal influences), while the greater frequency of labial carcinoma among men (22.7 %) suggests that pipe smoking may be a predisposing factor, as has also been suggested by Burkhardt and Seifert (1977). Pindborg (1977) too, has pointed out that labial carcinoma is 9 to 20 times more frequent among men than women in several European countries.

Pindborg and co-workers (1972), and more recently Kramer and collaborators (1978) have advocated the differentiation of sublingual keratosis from the other forms of oral leukoplakia. Carcinomatous change was detected in 27 % of 63 patients with leukoplakia of the floor of the mouth (sublingual keratosis), and follow-up studies of 29 patients for 1–19 years revealed malignant transformation in 24.1 % of cases. We observed a considerably lower incidence (9.7 %) of malignant transformation in our patients with leukoplakia of the floor of the mouth. Pindborg (1978) states that this type of leukoplakia is 2 to 4 times more frequent among women than men, but we have failed to substantiate this finding.

The clinical type of leukoplakia seems to be important in relation to malignant change. We demonstrated in earlier studies (Bánóczy and Csiba 1972) a correlation between clinical type and histological appearance. According to Pindborg et al. (1963), Roed-Petersen (1971), as well as Kramer and co--workers (1978), speckled leukoplakia is more liable to malignant transformation than the type they called homogeneous. Roed-Petersen (1971) observed malignant transformation in 9.1 % of speckled lesions, against only 1.3 % in other types. As the clinical type that we call "erosive" can be regarded as identical with the one designated by Danish authors as "speckled", we agree that this particular type is especially at risk. In our follow-up studies cancer development was observed in 28 % of erosive and 4.6 % of verrucous leukoplakias; an observation which, apart from substantiating the major hazard of malignant change in the erosive type, validifies our three-type classification. Of the carcinomas observed in our follow-up studies 74 % arose from erosive leukoplakia and 26 % from verrucous leukoplakia. This is unequivocal evidence of a close correlation between clinical type and malignant change, stated also by others (Seifert and Burkhardt 1979, Burkhardt 1980).

CHAPTER II

THE ROLE OF ETIOLOGICAL FACTORS

The 520 cases of leukoplakia included in the follow-up study were examined for causal factors, the percentage distribution of which is shown in Table 10.

It was found that 83% of the patients were smokers, and in 31.9% there were indications of the etiological involvement of mechanical factors. Thirteen per cent of the patients were alcoholics, 2.5% had a history of syphilis, 3% showed extreme differences in electric potential, and 13.5% had candidiasis. Multiple etiological factors were demonstrated in 195 (37.5%) of the 520 cases, while in 22 cases (4.2%) including 18 women, no obvious factor was found.

Of the 31 patients who developed carcinoma from leukoplakia 24 (77%) were smokers. Mechanical irritation (45%), alcoholism (33%), syphilis (10%), electric potential difference (15%) and candidiasis (65%) were more frequent in cases which underwent malignant change. A possible causal factor was lacking in only one case of carcinoma (3.2%). More than half (52%; 16 patients) of the malignant transformations arose in leukoplakias ascribed to multifactorial etiology.

Table 10

Percentage distribution of etiological factors within the groups of patients with leukoplakia and carcinoma*

Etiological factors	Leukoplakia %	Carcinoma %
Smoking habit	83.0	77.0
Mechanical irritation	31,9	45.0
Alcohol addiction	13.0	33.0
Syphilis	2.5	10.0
Differences in electric potential	3.0	19.3
Candida albicans infection	13.5	65.0
No obvious causal factor	4.2	3.2
Several causal factors	37.5	52.0

* In some cases several etiological factors could be demonstrated.

THE ETIOLOGICAL IMPORTANCE OF SMOKING HABITS

The etiological role of smoking in the development of oral leukoplakia and in its malignant transformation has been analyzed from two points of view, i.e. its potential to enhance keratinization and its carcinogenic effects.

Cytological investigations

Most authors engaged in follow-up studies of large groups of patients with leukoplakia have agreed on the etiological role of smoking (Mela and Mongini 1966*a*, Pindborg et al. 1968), but Fasske et al. (1959*a*, *b*) have questioned its importance and have classified a substantial number of their leukoplakias as idiopathic. Many clinical, cytological and histological studies have suggested that a smoking habit accounts for hyperkeratosis of the oral mucosa in predisposed individuals (Lewis 1955, Bánóczy 1962, Pindborg and Renstrup 1963, Knychalska-Karwan 1965*a*, *c*, Smith et al. 1970, Lainson and Mackenzie 1975, Rubinstein et al., Gupta et al. 1980), and that stopping the habit in the early stage of change may result in remission (Prinz 1928, Balogh 1956, Waldron 1965, L. Sugár and Bánóczy 1969).

Ayre (1957) established that smoking altered the cytological appearance of the oral mucosa, and that the degree of keratinization was inversely related to the number of cigarettes smoked daily. Calonius (1961) reported a significant increase in gingival keratinization in male habitual smokers. Hahn (1962*a*) observed a quantitative increase of acidophilic cells, and a reduction in their nuclear size. On the other hand, Wrubel and Scopp (1962) failed to detect significant differences between smears taken from the hard palate and buccal mucosa of men two weeks before adopting a smoking habit and two weeks after having stopped it. Zimmermann and Zimmermann (1965) observed a quantitative increase of acidophilic cells from the buccal mucosa of smokers.

The cytological technique developed by Papanicolaou and Traut in 1943 was selected by us as a simple and reproducible procedure for the study of alterations in oral keratinization that might be related to smoking.

The study of any pathological alterations was in fact preceded by observation of the normal cytological characteristics of the intact oral mucosa, and of the factors which influence it. Such investigations were pioneered by Weinmann in 1940, who used smears stained by the method of Ernst and Gram to identify the keratinization pattern in different parts of the mouth. Later Miller and co-workers (1951) and Montgomery (1951) employed the Papanicolaou technique, which made possible the classification of oral epithelial cells into six groups according to the degree of keratinization, as indicated by their taking on blue, red or yellow stain. This classification has been

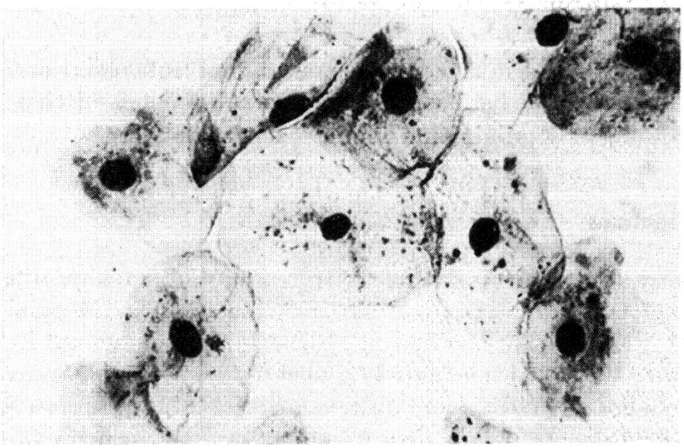

Fig. 9. Cytological appearance of normal buccal mucosa. The desquamated superficial epithelial cells have small, pyknotic nuclei, and some contain one or more keratohyaline granules. Papanicolaou's stain, ×340

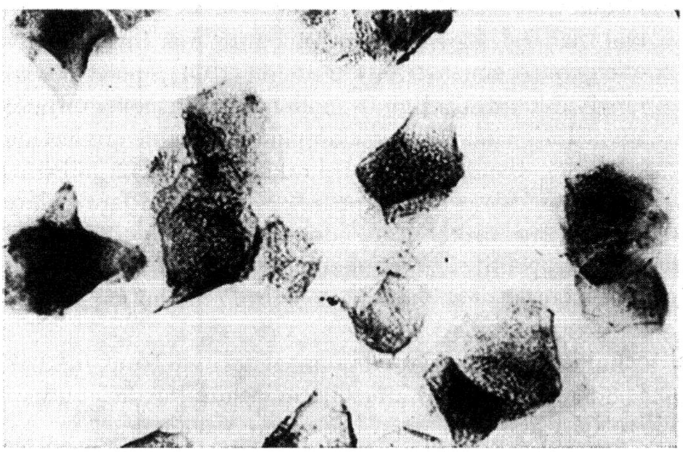

Fig. 10. Cytological appearance of normal palatal mucosa. The superficial epithelial cells are fully keratinized, without nuclei. Papanicolaou's stain, ×340

applied in my related investigations (Bánóczy 1958, 1960*a*, 1961*a*, 1969*a*, 1970; Figs 9 and 10). Unlike the authors cited above Hahn (1962*a*) distinguished nine keratinization types among cells from intact oral mucosa. These and related studies have led to the following conclusions:

1. The cytological appearance of the intact oral mucosa is not uniform, it varies with the anatomical site and functional status of the cells. In smears taken from the hard palate cells are almost exclusively of keratinized "yellow" type, the gingiva and dorsum of the tongue yields a mixed population of keratinized and non-keratinized cells, while such cells are scarcely seen in smears from the buccal region, floor of the mouth, and ventral surface of the tongue (see Figs 9 and 10).

2. The cytological picture may be influenced by age, sex, hormonal changes and local factors. Among the latter smoking habit and wearing of dentures are of major importance.

Evaluation of the etiological importance of smoking was made from a comparative study of the cytology of oral mucosa in smokers and non-smokers (Bánóczy 1962) of both sexes. The subjects were 20 to 60 years old, and had macroscopically intact oral mucous membrane. Smokers with a visible leukoplakia were excluded from the study. All smokers had their daily intake of at least 10 cigarettes. Pipe smokers were not included in the study, for most subjects with this habit exhibit visible hyperkeratosis of the oral mucosa.

The groups of male and female, smokers and non-smokers contained 25 subjects each, giving a total 100 persons who were examined as follows: In the morning the mouth was rinsed and mucosal scrapings were taken with a metal spatula from three sites: buccal mucosa, along the occlusal line, anterior dorsum of the tongue and antero-lateral part of the hard palate.

Table 11

Counts of keratinized cells in different oral sites of leukoplakia in patients with and without smoking habit

Sites and staining of cells		Women		Men	
		Smokers	Non-smokers	Smokers	Non-smokers
Buccal mucosa	blue	78	70	78	70
	red	20	27	20	25
	yellow	2	3	2	5
Tongue	blue	47	35	40	35
	red	28	22	36	26
	yellow	25	43	24	39
Hard palate	blue	10	8	9	8
	red	15	40	40	20
	yellow	57	77	51	72

The results are shown in Table 11, as averages from findings in the 25 subjects in each group.

Separate investigation of the sexes was prompted by earlier observations of sex differences in the keratinization pattern of the oral mucosa (Bánóczy 1958, 1960*a*). These differences were also obvious in the present studies. Mathematical-statistical *evaluation revealed a significant increase of keratinized cells in the epithelium of the tongue and hard palate of both male and female smokers* (Table 12).

An increase in the number of keratinized cells above the normal average can be equated with the clinical evidence that grossly visible hyperkeratosis of oral mucosa may arise in habitual smokers. It follows that smoking enhances the keratinization potential of oral epithelial cells, and cytological evidence of this can be obtained long before its clinical manifestation. The controversial findings of Wrubel and Scopp (1961) were based on smears taken only two weeks after stopping the smoking habit. As epithelial turnover in oral mucosa takes 16–23 days depending on the site (Meyer 1967, Meyer et al. 1960), two weeks was obviously too short a time to permit the superficial cytological expression of changes associated with the withdrawal of smoking.

Observations by ourselves and others have unequivocally permitted the conclusion that smoking may give way to hyperkeratotic changes in oral muco-

Table 12

Mathematical-statistical evaluation of differences between keratinized cell counts in three oral sites of leukoplakia in patients with and without a smoking habit

Oral site		Non-smokers $\bar{X}_1$	Smokers $\bar{X}_2$	t	p	Degree of significance
				[48]		
Women	Buccal mucosa	2	3	0.54	0.50–0.60	not significant
	Tongue	25	43	2.01	0.05	significant
	Hard palate	57	77	2.5	0.02	significant
Men	Buccal mucosa	2	5	1.34	0.10–0.20	not significant
			Analysis of the same difference with the Litchfield–Wilcoxon test showed a significant difference at 95% probability level.			
	Tongue	24	39	3.9	< 0.001	highly significant
	Hard palate	51	72	2.05	< 0.05	significant

sa, which in due course may be expressed clinically as oral leukoplakia. The development and site of the lesion may be influenced to different degrees by qualitative and/or quantitative changes in the smoking habit, and by individual disposition. In the group of patients with leukoplakia observed by Wilsch et al. (1978), 75% of the subjects were smokers; among these, the average cigarette consumption was higher, and the smoking period was longer compared to smokers without leukoplakia. Roed-Petersen et al. (1972) concluded from multivariant computer analysis that sex differences observed in the incidence of the leukoplakia were due to the dissimilar smoking habits of men and women.

Mehta et al. (1961, 1969*a*, *c*) established that the site of leukoplakia depends among other things on the type of smoking habit, as well as on the quality and quantity of the tobacco consumed. The habit of smoking "bidi", which is wide spread in India, accounts for the development of leukoplakia chiefly at the commissure or buccal mucosa, while cheroot smoking, much preferred in Denmark, is associated with leukoplakia of the floor of the mouth (Pindborg et al. 1972).

Histological examinations

The possible relationship between smoking habits and the histological characteristics of leukoplakia has received little attention. Orr (1933), Balendra (1949) and Marsden (1960) agreed that Eastern Indians with chewing habits generally exhibited epithelial hyperplasia as the predominant histological change, but subsequent findings have been more equivocal. Pindborg and collaborators (1964) established that microscopically the epithelial lesions varied with the type of smoking habit, even if their clinical appearances were similar. Meyer and his co-workers (1967) also observed different epithelial changes in tobacco chewers. Mehta et al. (1969*a*, *b*, *c*) and Pindborg et al. (1971) reported that in India, the microscopic appearance of oral leukoplakia varies with the type of smoking and chewing habit prevalent in different regions.

Opinions have also been divergent on the influence of smoking on cancer development from leukoplakia (Cawson 1957). Comparison of the incidence of dysplasia and carcinoma in patients with leukoplakia, who either chewed tobacco or not, revealed no significant difference between the two categories (Smith et al. 1970). Roed-Petersen and Pindborg (1973) arrived at the same conclusion in longitudinal studies. Balogh and Huszár (1962) frequently observed a mild form of leukoplakia, but did not find a single case of malignant transformation among gypsies notorius for non-stop tobacco chewing. Cooke (1967) also held the view that a distinction should be made between keratosis due to smoking, and dyskeratotic leukoplakia.

As studies of any possible correlation between smoking habits and the type of histological change had not previously been carried out in a European population, a comparative analysis of groups of Danish and Hungarian patients with leukoplakia was launched to obtain more information on the problem (Roed-Petersen et al. 1973). Comparison was facilitated by the year-long collaboration of the Danish and Hungarian investigators in the W. H. O. Collaborating Centre for Oral Precancerous Lesions and by the standarization of data and sample collection and processing methods. It was also expected that the comparative study might throw light on the possible impact of geographical factors on interrelationships between smoking habits and the incidence of leukoplakia (Mehta et al. 1969*a*, *c*, Pindborg et al. 1972).

A total of 345 and 184 biopsies from Danish and Hungarian subjects, respectively, were included in the study. Tobacco chewers were excluded from both groups, which thus consisted predominantly of cigarette smokers, but included some cheroot, cigar or pipe smokers. Occasional smokers were included with non-smokers. Men numbered 193 (55.6 %) and 153 (83.2 %), women 154 (44.4 %) and 31 (16.8 %) in the respective Danish and Hungarian groups.

Tables 13–16 show the relationship between smoking habit and four types of histological change, keratinization, thickness of epithelium, epithelial

Table 13

Distribution of keratotic changes in smokers and non-smokers in groups of Danish and Hungarian patients with leukoplakia

Type of keratinization	Non-smokers		Smokers		Totals	
	No.	%	No.	%	No.	%
Danish group (n = 345)						
hyperorthokeratosis	23	52.3	118	39.2	141	40.9
hyperparakeratosis	13	29.5	123	40.9	136	39.4
both	8	18.2	60	19.9	68	19.7
Totals	44	100.0	301	100.0	345	100.0
Hungarian group (n =184)						
hyperorthokeratosis	7	50.0	64	37.6	71	38.6
hyperparakeratosis	5	35.7	80	47.1	85	46.2
both	2	14.3	26	15.3	28	15.2
Totals	14	100.0	170	100.0	184	100.0

Table 14

Thickness of epithelium in smokers and non-smokers in groups of Danish and Hungarian patients with leukoplakia

Thickness of epithelium	Non-smokers		Smokers		Totals	
	No.	%	No.	%	No.	%
Danish group (n = 345)						
hyperplasia	14	31.8	70	23.3	84	24.4
atrophy	17	38.7	110	36.5	127	36.8
both	6	13.6	50	16.6	56	16.2
normal	7	15.9	71	23.6	78	22.6
Totals	44	100.0	301	100.0	345	100.0
Hungarian group (n = 184)						
hyperplasia	8	57.2	112	65.9	120	65.3
atrophy	4	28.6	24	14.1	28	15.2
both	1	7.1	11	6.5	12	6.5
normal	1	7.1	23	13.5	24	13.0
Totals	14	100.0	170	100.0	184	100.0

Table 15

Degree of connective tissue inflammation in smokers and non-smokers in groups of Danish and Hungarian patients with leukoplakia

Inflammatory change	Non-smokers		Smokers		Total	
	No.	%	No.	%	No.	%
Danish group (n = 345)						
absent or slight	32	72.7	186	61.8	218	63.2
medium or severe	12	27.3	115	38.2	127	36.8
Totals	44	100.0	301	100.0	345	100.0
Hungarian group (n = 184)						
absent or slight	11	78.6	126	74.1	137	74.5
medium or severe	3	21.4	44	25.9	47	25.5
Total	14	100.0	170	100.0	184	100.0

Table 16

Epithelial dysplasia incidence in smokers and non-smokers in groups of Danish and Hungarian patients with leukoplakia

Epithelial dysplasia	Non-smokers		Smokers		Total	
	No.	%	No.	%	No.	%
Danish group (n = 345)						
present	6	13.6	47	15.6	53	15.4
absent	38	86.4	254	84.4	292	84.6
Totals	44	100.0	301	100.0	345	100.0
Hungarian group (n = 184)						
present	6	42.9	47	27.6	53	28.8
absent	8	57.1	123	72.4	131	71.2
Totals	14	100.0	170	100.0	184	100.0

dysplasia and connective tissue inflammation (Roed-Petersen et al. 1973). Mathematical–statistical analysis revealed no significant difference between smokers and non-smokers in any category of change ($p < 0.5$).

Certain trends were nevertheless obvious in both groups of patients. The keratotic change was predominantly a hyperorthokeratosis in non-smokers, and hyperparakeratosis among smokers (Table 13). Similarly moderate to severe connective tissue inflammation was more frequent among smokers than non-smokers.

It was concluded that *the degree of keratinization, epithelial thickness, epithelial dysplasia and inflammation did not differ significantly between smokers and non-smokers* in either the Hungarian or the Danish groups (Roed-Petersen et al. 1973).

Several authors (Einhorn and Wersäll 1967, Roed-Petersen 1971, Gangadharan and Paymaster 1971, Bánóczy and L. Sugár 1972, Bánóczy 1977) have found a greater prevalence of cancer development among non-smoking than smoking patients with leukoplakia. This accords well with the observation (Table 16) that the incidence of dysplasia was near identical among the Danish smokers and non-smokers, and even higher among non-smokers (42.9 %) than smokers in the Hungarian group. However, the relatively low number of cases involved permits no definitive conclusions. In contrast, Silverman and Griffith (1972) reported a positive correlation between smoking habit and cancer incidence in a longitudinal study of 174 patients with oral carcinoma, among whom the risk of developing a second primary malignancy seemed to increase if the habit was maintained.

Finally, consideration should be given to the observation of Mehta et al. (1969*c*) that different regions of the oral mucosa respond differently to irritation by smoking, and their microscopic changes vary accordingly.

THE ETIOLOGICAL IMPORTANCE OF MECHANICAL FACTORS

Several investigators including myself (Hetessy 1960*a*, *b*, Bánóczy and L. Sugár 1972, Kövesi and Bánóczy 1973, Lelkes 1973, Bánóczy 1974) have indicated that mechanical factors may either alone or in combination with other factors, cause a local irritation of the oral mucosa. Lelkes (1973) found a correlation between the state of dentition and the incidence of leukoplakia; among 362 patients with leukoplakia 28% had neglected teeth. The etiological involvement of mechanical factors may be substantiated by demonstrating a relationship between the site of leukoplakia and the area of physical irritation. Therefore sharp-edged teeth (sharp cusps, broken crowns or roots), or sharp-edged bridges and partial or complete dentures were examined for their potentially irritant effects.

Mechanical factors that might cause physical irritation were found in 166 (31.9%) of the 520 patients. The type of mechanical irritant is shown in Table 17. The frequency of sharp-edged (or broken) natural teeth and partial or complete prostheses was roughly similar. The proportion of leukoplakias associated with a sharp-edged dental bridge was very low.

Subsequently we examined the extent of the relationship between the use of a partial or complete dental prosthesis and the incidence of oral mucosal lesions, with special regard to their site (Tables 18 and 19).

Of the 520 patients with leukoplakia 96 (18.4%) had complete upper and lower dentures and 78 (15%) partial dentures. The site of leukoplakia could

Table 17

Distribution of different types of mechanical irritation in patients with leukoplakia

Mechanical irritants	Cases	
	No.	%
Sharp-edged natural tooth	54	32.6
Sharp-edged dental bridge	11	6.5
Complete denture	49	29.4
Partial denture	52	31.5
Totals	166	100.0

Table 18

Frequency of mechanical irritation among patients with leukoplakia wearing dentures

Denture	Leukoplakia cases			
	related		unrelated	
	to irritation			
	No.	%	No.	%
Complete	49	51.0	47	49.0
Partial	52	66.6	26	33.4
Totals	101		73	

Table 19

Relationship between the site of leukoplakia and the use of a prosthesis

Site of lesion	Patients wearing				Total	
	complete		partial			
	denture					
	No.	%	No.	%	No.	%
Buccal mucosa	32	65.3	39	75.0	71	70.3
Alveolar ridge	17	34.7	13	25.0	30	29.7
Totals	49	100.0	52	100.0	101	100.0

be related to the prosthesis in 51 and 66% of the cases with complete and partial dentures, respectively. Statistical analysis revealed that an association with leukoplakia was significantly greater ($p < 0.05$) among patients with a partial prosthesis than among those with complete dentures.

The sites of leukoplakias that had an obvious relationship with mechanical irritation by a dental prosthesis are shown in Table 19.

It follows that *the site of leukoplakias related to such mechanical irritation was usually the buccal mucosa, less often the alveolar ridge, and, occasionally, the hard palate* (see Fig. 5). Differences in site between leukoplakias related to the use of either a partial or complete dental prosthesis were not significant statistically ($0.3 > p > 0.1$).

The occurrence of hyperkeratosis of the alveolar ridge, a frequent result of wearing unsatisfactory dentures was analyzed separately. Among the 520 patients 34 had a lesion on the alveolar ridge; of these, 30 (88.3%) wore a denture, and four (11.7 %) did not. All these denture-wearers were found to have an imperfectly fitting prosthesis. Patients with leukoplakia who had a perfectly fitting denture did not had lesions on the alveolar ridge, even if they were habitual smokers.

The etiological importance of mechanical factors in oral leukoplakia has received little attention from investigators engaged in the follow-up of large groups of patients. Lelkes (1973) agreed with us that the main site of leukoplakia related to mechanical irritation was the middle zone of the buccal mucosa, which showed hyperkeratotic change in 57 % if his cases. This is the common site at which the oral mucosa may become wedged between the teeth or irritated by sharp-edged, broken teeth or imperfectly fitting prostheses. Lelkes reported that after remedial dental treatment, 38 % of his patients with leukoplakia recovered, 47 % showed improvement and only 15 % did not respond. Vándor (1969) also observed spontaneous remission in some cases of leukoplakia after correction of the dentition.

It is remarkable that certain authors (Tiecke and Bernier 1954, Mackenzie and Miles 1973) have questioned the role of mechanical factors in the malignant transformation of oral leukoplakia, claiming that chronic mechanical irritation cannot in itself give rise to malignancy. The etiological involvement of mechanical irritation was demonstrable in 45 % of our cases of oral carcinoma arising from leukoplakia, i.e. in a considerably greater proportion than in the group of unaltered leukoplakias. This strongly suggests that mechanical factors play some part in malignant transformation. Similar observations have been reported by Bredy (1955) and Haym (1961).

THE ETIOLOGICAL IMPORTANCE OF DIFFERENCES IN ELECTRICAL POTENTIAL

It has long been known that differences in electrical potential may arise in the mouth between different metal fillings and metal restorations. The symptoms elicited by the potential difference can be divided into two main types; (*a*) subjective complaints that follow immediately upon placement of the metal restoration, such as metallic taste, and (*b*) subjective symptoms or signs that develop later, such as chronic inflammation of oral mucosa and neuralgic pain.

Investigations into this problem date back to the end of the last century. Chase in 1879 incriminated various metals in tooth destruction. Electric activity due to potential differences in the mouth was first measured by Lain (1933) and later by many others such as Simsa (1955), Denier (1955) and Rheinwald et al. (1954). Opinions have been divergent on the conditions of generation, and on the nature of the electric current. Most authors have attributed it to the formation of a galvanic cell (Hollander et al. 1933, Lain 1933, Solomon and Reinhard 1934, Balban 1936, Touraine and Baudouin 1937), but recently the role of bioelectric forces has been emphasized (Schriever and Diamond 1952, Rheinwald 1956). In Hungary the bioelectric effect has been investigated *in vitro* by Tarnai and Záray (1953*a*, *b*), who measured potential differences between certain metals, relative to a calomel electrode placed in saliva.

Injury to the oral mucosa by electrical potential difference between metals has been reported by several investigators (Kiss 1955, Melczer and Kiss 1956, Kuffer and Rouchon 1967). Ullmann studied the problem as long ago as 1932, in a group of 580 patients with leukoplakia, of which three developed oral carcinoma.

In previous studies along this line, we observed a considerable improvement of chronic diseases of the oral mucosa, above all of leukoplakia, after the removal of metal restorations that accounted for high potential differences (Inovay and Bánóczy 1960*a*, *b*).

In the present study, the electrical potential was determined only in the cases with differing metal restoration, if (*i*) no other etiological factor was found, or (*ii*) the lesion did not respond to treatment.

Of the 520 patients, 16 (3%) had potential differences exceeding 50 mV, and of these six (37.5%) developed carcinoma (19.3% of the total number of carcinomas), *It seems that large differences in electric potential may promote the malignant transformation of oral leukoplakia.*

The age and sex distribution of patients with leukoplakia and high electric potential differences is shown in Table 20.

The proportion of males and females was similar but of the six carcinoma patients with high potential difference five were women. As to concurrent etio-

Table 20

Age and sex distribution of patients with leukoplakia and electrical potential differences (figures in brackets refer to cancer development from leukoplakia)

Age (years)	Men	Women	Total
30–39	1 (1)	3 (1)	4
40–49	—	—	—
50–59	5	2 (2)	7
60–69	2	1 (1)	3
>70	1	1 (1)	2
Totals	9	7	16

Table 21

Length of observation periods

Observation periods in years	No. of cases
>1 – <5	7
>5 – <10	3
>10 – <20	5
>20	1
Totals	16

logical factors, all the men were smokers, and of the seven women one smoked. Three female patients with cancer developing from leukoplakia had iron-deficiency anaemia, and also glossitis as one part of the Plummer–Vinson syndrome. In two females with potential difference there was no indication of any other etiological factor. It should be noted that all five females with carcinoma had the tumour on the tongue, while the male patient, developed carcinoma in a buccal leukoplakia.

Table 21 shows the length of the observation periods. In all six cases of carcinoma leukoplakia had been present for more than 10 years, which again points to the importance of the time factor.

The findings in control examinations after exchange of metal restorations and/or surgical treatment are shown in Table 22.

The number of cases of major differences in electrical potential encountered in our follow-up study is too small to permit definitive conclusions, but clinical observations suggest that exchange of the metal restoration responsible

Table 22

Findings of control examinations after treatment

Treatment methods	Improvement	Spread (carcinoma)
Exchange of metal restorations	5	–
Exchange of metal restorations + surgical treatment	2	3
Surgical treatment without exchange of metal restorations	3	3
Totals	10	6

for generating the current in the early stage of leukoplakia may result in reversal of the lesion. However, a combination of exchange of restorations and surgical treatment will fail to arrest the change if it has been present for at least a decade.

THE ROLE OF INFLAMMATORY AND ATROPHIC CHANGES OF THE ORAL MUCOUS MEMBRANE IN THE PATHOGENESIS OF LEUKOPLAKIA

Atrophy of epithelium on the tongue and lip as a sequel to recurrent acute or chronic inflammation of the mucosa has been shown to promote the development of leukoplakia (Vándor 1969). The mechanism underlying such changes is not infrequently endogenous. Szodoray (1963) and Maskillejson (1969) regarded photosensitive cheilitis as a precancerous state, and Vonkei and J. Sugár (1965) classified the chronic forms of cheilitis as facultative precancerous changes that predispose to the development of frank precancerosis, leukoplakia. Lőrinczy (1956) suggested that two frequent pathological conditions of the oral mucosa, chronic erythematous stomatitis and chronic catarrhal stomatitis, are important pathogenetic factors in oral leukoplakia. Erythematous inflammation causes atrophy of the lingual papillae, which then fail to regenerate; this change is termed "lingua geographica" or "geographic tongue" if it appears in patches, and "mirror tongue" if it involves the entire surface. The latter change is also known as Hunter–Möller glossitis if it occurs in association with pernicious anaemia, and it may also be found as a part of the Plummer–Vinson syndrome, which is an expression of microcytic, iron-deficient anaemia. Chronic catarrhal inflammation is associated with enhanced keratinization of the filiform papillae, and its clinical appearance is hardly distinguishable from leukoplakia. Also, it has long been known that the Plummer–Vinson syndrome (Paterson–Kelly syndrome) may be a precancerous state (Hertz 1956, Weisberger 1957, Kuhn and Ravasz 1964). In Scandinavia the syndrome is positively correlated with oral or oesophageal carcinoma among female patients (Clemmesen 1965). Development of leukoplakia (L. Sugár et al. 1975) or carcinoma (Sharp and Bullock 1958, Lentrodt and Luhr 1970) in glossitis mediana rhombica has been observed. We therefore examined in great detail patients with lesions of "geographic tongue" or migratory glossitis, Hunter–Möller glossitis, glossitis with the Plummer–Vinson syndrome, and glossitis mediana rhombica.

Migratory glossitis*

In 1881 Unna described a lesion of the tongue which he called "exfoliatio areata linguae". This appeared as red patches of varying shape and size, the terms "wandering rash", "erythema migrans" (Prinz 1927, Halperin et al. 1953), and "benign glossitis migrans" (Cooke 1962) were adopted in the Anglo-Saxon medical literature, together with other names that refer to the map-like appearance of the tongue, such as "lingua geographica" (L. Sugár 1959) or "geographic tongue" (Meskin et al. 1963, Zegarelli et al. 1963, Richardson 1968). Several authors, however, still prefer the designation "exfoliatio areata linguae et mucosae oris" (Schuermann 1958, Strassburg and Knolle 1968, Kuffer et al. 1971).

Various investigators give the incidence of migratory glossitis as from 0.28 to 14.4% (McCarthy 1941, Halperin et al. 1953, Rahamimoff and Muhsam 1957, Meskin et al. 1963, Redman et al. 1966, Richardson 1968, Redman 1970, Axell 1975, Chosack et al. 1977). Opinions have varied as to its etiology. Some authors such as Greither (1955), Zegarelli and co-workers (1969) and Shafer and collaborators (1974) have called it a congenital defect, while others regard it as either an acute inflammatory, or a chronic post-erythematous state (lingua geographica, Cooke 1962, Lőrinczy-Landgraf 1968). Factors which influence the course of the condition, as well as the necessity for and form of treatment are also controversial. Follow-up studies of migratory glossitis in a large group of patients (39 subjects) have been reported by only one author (Cooke 1962).

In an attempt to reconcile conflicting opinions on the clinical and pathological aspects of the condition, and to make an objective approach to the subjective complaints and cancerophobia of many of the affected patients, we made a restrospective study of 70 cases of migratory glossitis seen in the Clinic of Maxillo-Facial Surgery and Dentistry, Dental Faculty of Semmelweis University Medical School, Budapest, from 1963 to 1972. Some of the patients were sent to the clinic by their family doctor because of the lingual lesion, some came without referral because of pain which had been present for either a short or a long time, and which various doctors had failed to treat. The purpose of the retrospective study was to obtain more information on the etiology, clinical and histological appearance, and course of the condition, as well as its response to treatment.

The *age and sex distribution* of the patients is shown in Table 23. The group comprised 46 women and 24 men. Thus females predominated (65.7%), and the female/male ratio was approximately 2:1. Half of the patients were either

* Excerpted with permission from Oral Surg. Oral Med. Oral Pathol. **39**: 113–121, 1975; copyrighted by The C. V. Mosby Company, St. Louis, Missouri U.S.A.

Table 23

Age and sex distribution of patients with migratory glossitis

Age (years)	Men	Women	Total
–9	1	3	4
10–19	1	2	3
20–29	5	10	15
30–39	2	3	5
40–49	7	7	14
50–59	3	7	10
60–69	2	12	14
>70	3	2	5
Totals	24	46	70

20 to 29 years old, or more than 64 years old (34 cases). Subjects aged 30–39 years were few in number. Two-thirds of the patients of both sexes were older than 40 years.

The *duration of the disease* was understood as period of time between the recognition of the lesion (by patient or doctor) and presentation in the clinic (Table 24).

Nineteen patients had no knowledge whatever of their condition. A 4-year-old girl had had migratory glossitis since birth according to her mother (see Fig. 11). A 24-year-old male had known about the lesion for 20 years, and a female, aged 44, for 34 years.

The *case histories* were analyzed for familial prevalence, association with other disease(s), factors influencing the condition and the frequency of

Table 24

Duration of the disease

Years	Men	Women	Total
<1	6	16	22
>1– <5	8	11	19
>5–<10	1	2	3
>10	2	5	7
Patient unaware	7	12	19
Totals	24	46	70

subjective complaints. A familial prevalence was demonstrated in two cases; the sister and mother of one patient, and the sister of another had migratory glossitis.

Among associated conditions plicated tongue (Fig. 11) occurred in 9 instances, and fissured tongue (Fig. 12) in 5, i.e. lingual lesions other than migratory glossitis were present in 20.1 % of the patients. In addition, 4 patients had candidiasis and 2 had lichen planus. In several cases, migratory glossitis was a sequel to some other condition. Subjective complaints arose in one case after gastrectomy, and in three cases after drug therapy (Isonicid resp. Tetran). Analysis of the case history revealed an association with pregnancy in one case, and with "nervousness" in 8 cases (Fig. 13).

The *frequency of symptoms* is shown in Table 25. Many patients reported sensitivity to sour or spicy foods, and a few, chiefly of menopausal age, a spontaneous burning sensation of the tongue (see Fig. 12). Cancerophobia was frequent. Of the 70 patients 78.6 % had subjective symptoms, while 26 % of the women and 12.5 % of the men had no complaint: this sex difference was not statistically significant.

As to *clinical appearance*, hyperaemic spots due to destruction of the filiform papillae were usually present on the dorsum and lateral margins of the tongue (Fig. 14 and colour photo 5). The fungiform papillae were preserved

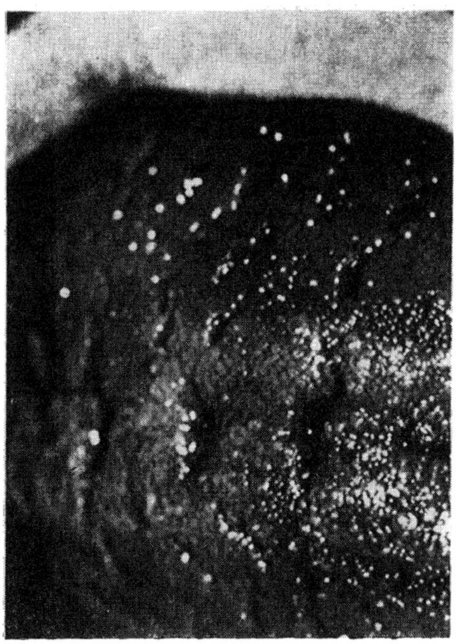

Fig. 11. Plicated tongue of a 4-year-old girl, with recurrent migratory glossitis. The child's mother reported that the lesion had been present since birth

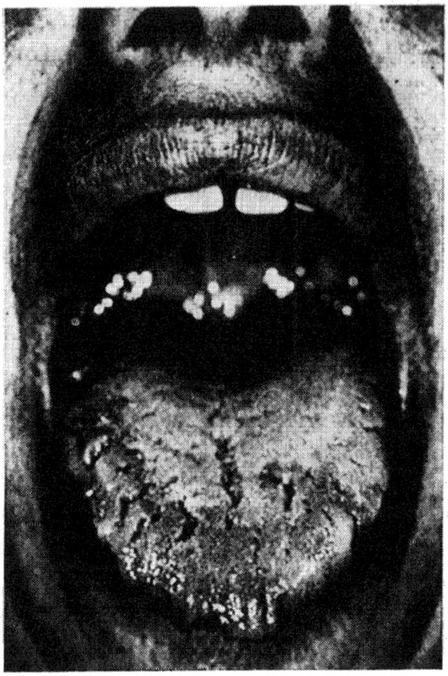

Fig. 12. Migratory glossitis plus fissured tongue in a 52-year-old female patient who presented with glossodynia. Note the impression left by the teeth on the margins of the swollen tongue

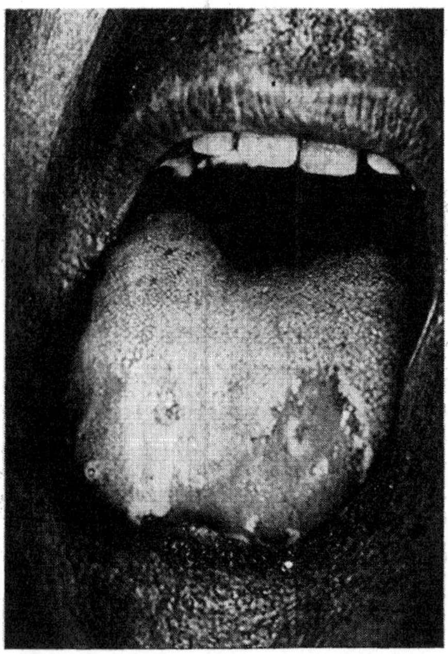

Fig. 13. Migratory glossitis (geographic tongue) in a 63-year-old male patient. At admission, the lesion had been present for one year, since the death of the patient's son. The subjective complaints improved after treatment for six months, but the symptoms persisted

Table 25

Frequency of symptoms

Symptoms	Men	Women	Total
Absent	4	11	15
Present	21	34	55
Totals	25	45	70

within the red patch, and around it the filiform papillae formed elevated collar (see colour photo 5). The red patches often changed their position within short periods. We found that the clinical symptoms tended to become more pronounced with progressive age (see Figs 13 and 14).

The results of laboratory examinations are shown in Table 26. Anaemia was suspectedin about half of the cases, but evidence of it was obtained only in one third (17% of all cases studied); 14.3% of the patients had candidiasis, and a few had gastric hyperacidity.

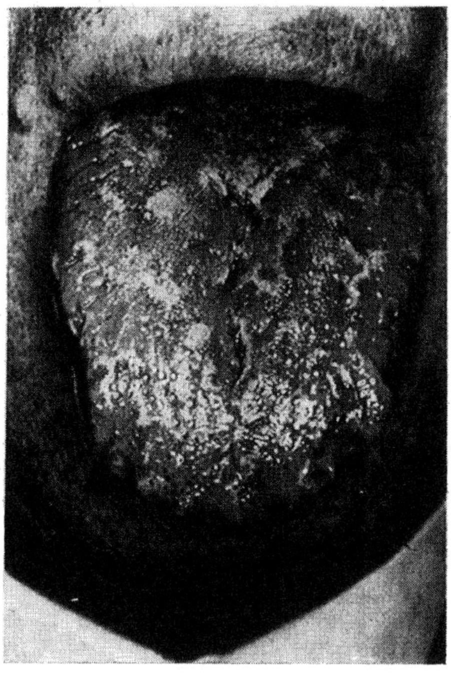

Fig. 14. Typical geographic tongue of a 68-year-old male patient with migratory glossitis. Note the collar-like thickening of the filiform papillae around the hyperaemic spots, and the impressions left by the teeth along the edge of the swollen, oedematous tongue

Histological examination was performed in 25 cases. Biopsies were always taken at the boundary between changed and normal tissues to include part of both.

On microscopic examination after staining with haematoxylin and eosin, the grossly normal mucosa showed minor oedema of the spinous cells, hyperchromatism of the basal cells, and a slight infiltration of the connective tissue by inflammatory cells. Superficial layers of the epithelium were parakeratinized. In the red patches acanthosis of the epithelium was associated with marked intra- and extracellular oedema. Aggregations of neutrophilic granulocytes appeared in the superficial layers of the epithelium (Monro's micro-abscess; Dawson 1969), and infiltration of the connective tissue was more pronounced than elsewhere. Rupture of the micro-abscesses at the surface accounted for desquamation of the parakeratotic layers, and subsequent denudation of the epithelial surface. In such areas the connective tissue papillae were covered by only a few layers of epithelial cells. Clinically the areas devoid of both filiform papillae and parakeratosis were at the centre of a red patch. The suprapapillary layer of the epithelium was infiltrated by lymphocytes, plasma cells and neutrophilic granulocytes. The elastic fibre of the connective tissue showed degenerative change (Fig. 15).

Desquamation of parakeratotic epithelial cells and the attendant micro-abscesses was followed by a reduction of inflammation, and by epithelial regeneration with parakeratosis.

The *methods of treatment* were selected with regard to the presence or absence of a complicating condition. Patients with candidiasis, anaemia, hyperacidity or hormonal disorders were treated accordingly. If the laboratory tests revealed no abnormality, local, symptomatic and vitamin therapy was employed, and nervous patients were treated with sedatives. Some

Table 26

Laboratory findings

Test	No. of cases
RBC count	
normal	23
anaemia	12
Isolation of *C. albicans*	
negative	13
positive	10
Gastric acidity	
normal	2
hyperacidity	4

Fig. 15. Microscopic appearance of migratory glossitis. The epithelium shows thickening and acanthosis in places. Note aggregation of neutrophilic granulocytes (Monro's abscess) in the superficial epithelium. The abscess is in process of detachment together with the parakeratotic epithelial layers. Note massive inflammatory cell infiltration in the subepithelial connective tissue. H. & E., ×125

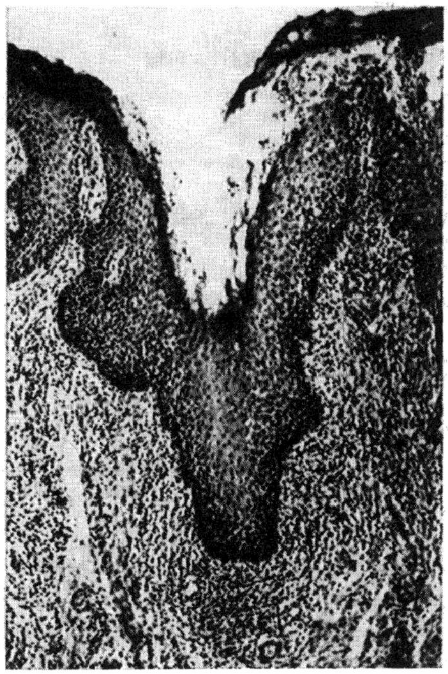

patients were given several forms of treatment either simultaneously or in accession. An objective evaluation of the therapeutic influence of sedatives was not possible, for most patients in need of them had taken them previously.

Patients were classified as "recovered" when papillae reappeared in the previously depapillated areas, or when subjective complaints subsided. Cases with an increase in subjective complaints or extension of the depapillated patches were classified as "worse".

As shown in Table 27, the treatments applied were successful in only 3.6 % of the cases. In the remainder they had no influence on either the lingual lesions or the subjective complaints.

The *period of observation* was the time interval between the first presentation and last re-examination of the patient. Of patients with migratory glossitis seen by the author 54 % were available for follow-up study.-The average length of the observation period was 2.8 years, but some patients were available for re-examination for 5 to 10 years. Their clinical state changed little but no malignant transformation occurred.

The age and sex distribution of patients with migratory glossitis corresponded with that observed of other authors (Prinz 1927, Halperin et al. 1953, Meskin et al. 1963). Most investigators reported a female/male ratio

Table 27

Methods and results of treatment

Method of treatment	Results of treatment			No. of patients not reexamined	Totals
	Healing	No change	Worse		
Local treatment	1	14	1	3	19
Vitamin A	—	9	2	—	11
Vitamin B	2	19	2	9	32
Vitamin C	—	4	—	2	6
Iron, Vitamin B_{12}	—	15	—	10	25
Antimycotic agent	—	9	—	3	12
Hormone(s)	—	1	2	—	2
Untreated	—	3	—	12	15
Totals	3	74	7	39	123

of 5:3 or 3:2. The greater frequency among women may be attributed to hormonal and/or psychological factors associated with the menopause since the number of female patients increased above 40 years of age. A sex ratio different to the above was reported by Rahamimoff and Muhsam (1957), and Cooke (1962) who found ratios of 3:4 and 1:1, respectively, but this may have been due to racial differences. Zegarelli et al. (1969) reported a frequent occurrence of this glossitis among children and young adults, but it was these age groups which were covered in their epidemiological study of a large unselected, symptom-free population while our patients had in most instances presented with symptoms they had already recognized. Most young patients seen by us had originally escorted older members of their family to the clinic, and the presence of similar lingual lesions in them was revealed only after the examination.

Several authors have observed the occurrence of migratory glossitis in small children. Rahamimoff and Muhsam (1957) found the condition in 14.4% of a group of more than 5,000 Israeli refugee children, aged 0 to 2 years. In our experience, intelligent and observant patients usually know about their lingual lesions from childhood.

The familial incidence of migratory glossitis was emphasized by Schuermann (1958), Kuffer and Brocheriou (1968). Turpin and Caratzali (1936) observed the condition retrospectively in three generations of one family, and described its occurrence in monozygous twins.

The frequency of the association between migratory glossitis and plicated tongue which, together with a fissured tongue, occurred in 20% of our cases, was estimated by Schuermann (1958) as 40–50%, but Farman (1976*a*) found an association with geographic tongue in only 1 of 24 cases of lingua fissurata detected in the course of screening 1,430 children. The role of nervous and psychological factors was pointed out by those who first described the condition during the second part of the last century (Gautier 1881, Unna 1881, Fox 1884). Aggravation of the symptoms by stress was observed by Cooke (1962) and Redman et al. (1966).

Kuffer et al. (1971) and Redman (1970), distinguished by their clinical appearances four stages of the lesion, which can also be defined histologically. Schuermann (1958) gave the time for a cycle of epithelial denudation and renewal as 2–10 days. Zegarelli et al. (1963) concluded from snapshots taken of the tongue every 15–30 min that the map-like appearance of the lesions may be completely changed within 2 h. The red patches were found to spread in a centrifugal direction, i.e. from the centre of the tongue towards its tip (Kuffer 1972) (see colour photo 5). In our experience, the depapillated patches tend to become larger and more pronounced with age (see Fig. 13); we agree with Lőrinczy (1956), and Lőrinczy-Landgraf (1947, 1958) that this is due to mucosal atrophy resulting from recurrent inflammation, and to failure of the filiform papillae to reappear in the atrophic areas.

Laboratory examinations revealed a frequent association between lingual lesions and disorders of the gastrointestinal tract. The occurrence of anaemia, or abnormal gastric secretion in some of our cases supports this association without indicating any obvious etiological relationship.

The histological appearance of migratory glossitis was described first by Gaston in 1902. Cooke (1962) interpreted the lesion as essentially inflammatory. Kuffer et al. (1971) distinguished four histological stages, i.e. epithelial inflammation with pustule formation, followed by desquamation and regeneration of the epithelium. Zegarelli et al. (1969) described a combination of hyperplasia and atrophy in the lesion. Our histological findings are in accord with these observations. The histological appearance of the lesion changed in relation to its clinical stage.

No specific therapy for migratory glossitis has as yet been proposed. Cooke (1962) and Balogh and Lelkes (1965) advocated the elimination of irritating factors (such as smoking), and recommended tranquillizers for nervous complaints. Several authors (Greither 1955, Strassborg and Knolle 1968, Kuffer et al. 1971, Hornstein 1976) held the view that no drug therapy is required, but that a positive psychological approach is imperative and the patient should be informed of the benign nature of the change. L. Sugár and colleagues (1975) recommended symptomatic treatment with mild adstringent mouth rinses, above all chamomile tea, and vitamin B therapy, but opposed the use of caustics. We agree with the elimination of irritants and mild symptomatic treatment, together with psychological reassurance of the patient.

We began longitudinal studies of migratory glossitis several years ago (Bánóczy et al. 1974, 1975), because there was insufficient information in the literature. *Malignant change has not been found since then in any case, irrespective of its duration.*

Lesions of the tongue in association with anaemia

A survey of the incidence of anaemia in all of our patients with leukoplakia was not possible, for blood tests had to be confined to the cases in which they were justified by subjective complaints or objective signs such as pallor of skin or mucous membranes, and/or atrophy of the lingual mucosa (mirror tongue) due to degeneration of the filiform papillae. The erythematous inflammation of the tongue, called Hunter–Möller glossitis, gives a smooth, glossy and bright red surface, while iron-deficiency anaemia produces a rather pale, pinkish-yellow discolouration. Objective complaints include burning of the tongue, gustatory impairment and pain during the ingestion of hot and/or strongly seasoned dishes. Persistence of the change for lack of adequate treatment may lead to the formation of cracks in the atrophic mucosa (fissured tongue), and if chronic irritation is also present, leukoplakia or even carcinoma may develop.

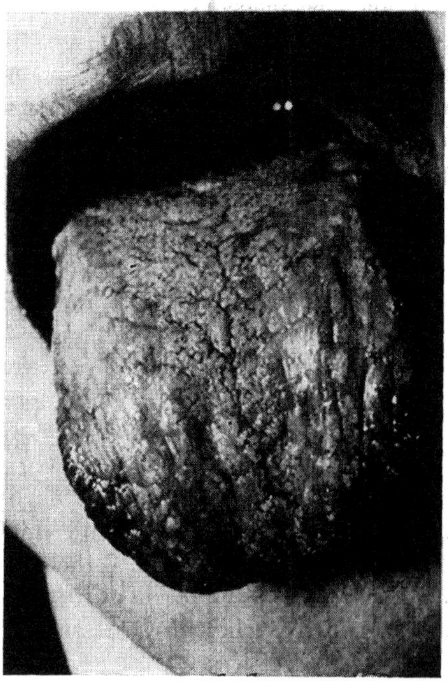

Fig. 16. Diffuse simple leukoplakia in a 44-year-old male patient on the dorsum of the tongue, which exhibits glossitis associated with the Plummer–Vinson syndrome

Among our patients four developed leukoplakia in a "mirror" tongue caused by anaemia, due to iron deficiency in three cases (two men and one woman, Fig. 16) and to pernicious anaemia in one case which had been known and treated for several years. In the latter case mechanical irritation by an ill-fitting denture, and a candidiasis (Fig. 17) may also have promoted the development of leukoplakia. Three patients with cancer development from leukoplakia, all women, aged, respectively 47, 58 and 61 years, at the onset of malignancy, had Plummer–Vinson syndrome. All three had leukoplakia on the tongue (Fig. 18 and colour photo 6), and two also on the alveolar ridge and floor of the mouth; in every case, the lesion was multicentric, large, and initially of the simplex-verrucous type. Later the verrucous lesions became ulcerated, and at this stage histological signs of malignancy were present. Because of their large size and location, the lesions were unsuitable for conservative treatment, and the patients failed to agree to surgical removal until it was too late and malignant change had occurred. Leukoplakia had been present for 31, 4 and 29 years, but the patients had no knowledge of their anaemia until the last 2–3 years.

These few cases should serve as a reminder of the greater risks attendant upon leukoplakia of the tongue in comparison to other sites, and of the importance of the early recognition and treatment of anaemia (Vándor 1978).

Median rhomboid glossitis

The first clinical descriptions of glossitis mediana rhombica were contributed by Brocq and Pautrier in 1914, and later by Lane (1924). The characteristic lesion, regarded as the major clinical sign, is a sharply circumscribed, oval or rhomboid, 1.5–3 cm long by 0.5–1 cm wide area of depapillated mucous membrane located in the midline of the tongue just anterior to the circumvallate papillae. The surface of the lesion is usually smooth, glossy, vivid or greyish red (colour photo 7), less often protruberant, uneven and verrucous (Fig. 19), (L. Sugár et al. 1975). The incidence of glossitis mediana rhombica varies between 0.15 and 3% (Halperin et al. 1954, Pindborg 1968, Richardson 1968, Zegarelli et al. 1969, Farman et al. 1977). It affects chiefly men (Martin and Howe 1941). Brocq and Pautrier (1914), Lane (1924) and uptil now many other authors (Sammet 1940, Hansen 1942, Kleiss 1949, Breitner 1950, Dechaume et al. 1958, Cooke 1962, Freedman et al. 1967, Pinkert 1967, Strassburg and Knolle 1968, Borello et al. 1972, Hornstein 1976) have classified it as a developmental abnormality that arises through the defective fusion of the two embryonic parts of the tongue with persistence of the tuberculum impar. Others (Loos and Hörbst 1934) have regarded it as a vascular naevus, because it contains dilated lymph vessels and capillaries. Recently Baughman and Charleston (1971) suggested the possibility of an inflamma-

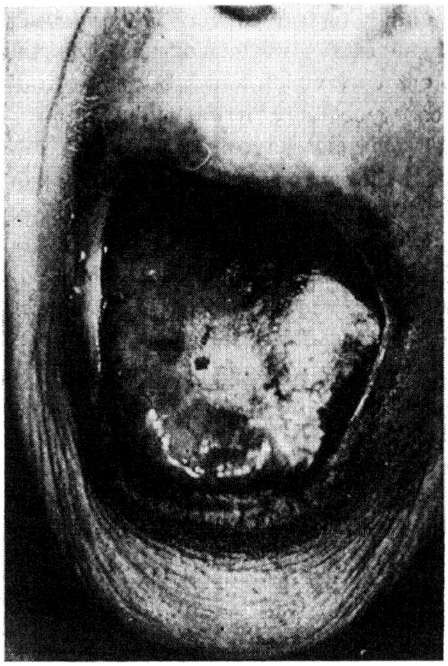

Fig. 17. Simple plus verrucous leukoplakia developed on the atrophic mirror tongue of a 72-year-old female patient with Hunter–Möller glossitis. The patient had worn an inadequate caoutchouc prosthesis, had oral candidiasis and had been treated for pernicious anaemia for several years

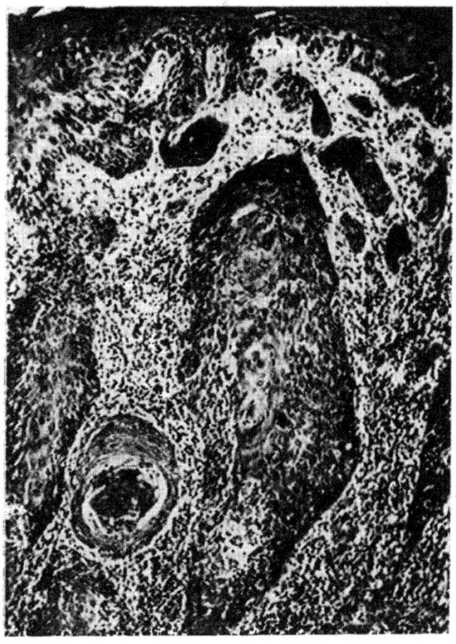

Fig. 18. Microscopic appearance of the lesion shown on colour photo 6: squamous cell carcinoma. H. & E., ×125

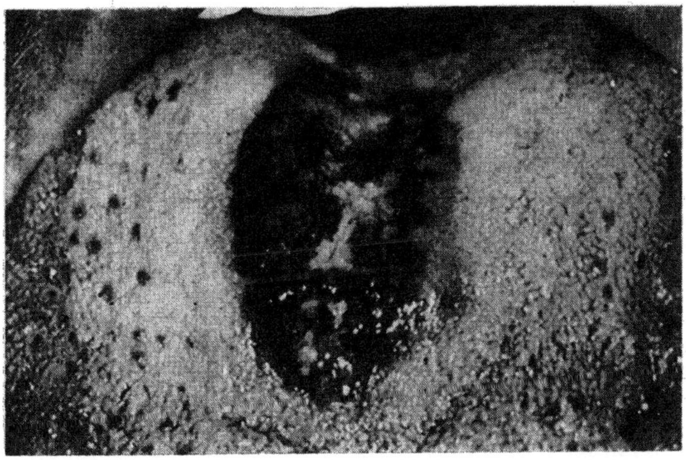

Fig. 19. Median rhomboid glossitis on the dorsum of the tongue of a 36-year-old female patient. The prominent lesion is depapillated. The patient wore a prosthesis; despite antimycotic treatment and excision the lesion recurred

tory or infectious origin, even a mycosis, a view supported by Pindborg (1973), Farman et al. (1975), Sugár et al. (1975), van der Waal et al. (1979) and Gupta et al. (1980). Farman (1976*b*) as well as Farman and Nutt (1976) observed an increased frequency of the condition among diabetics, and demonstrated histologically a microvascular degeneration.

Cooke (1962) and Pinkert (1967) reported a frequent association of glossitis mediana rhombica with cancerophobia. Engelstad (1941), Freedman et al. (1967), Lentrodt and Luhr (1970) pointed to frequent difficulties in the differential diagnosis of the lesion from carcinoma. Development of carcinoma from glossitis mediana rhombica has been reported by Sharp and Bullock (1958), Alshanetzky (1959), and Lentrodt and Luhr (1970).

As the etiology, pathogenesis and prognosis of the lesion are still uncertain, we analyzed by longitudinal study the clinical characteristics and course of cases of glossitis mediana rhombica encountered amongst our group of patients with leukoplakia.

Of the 520 patients in our follow-up study, 12 had glossitis mediana rhombica. This gives an incidence of 2.3% within this selected group, which is very high compared to the incidences observed by others in unselected populations. Of the 12 patients nine were men and three were women; this is in accord with other observations that the condition is prevalent in the males. The age and sex distribution are shown in Table 28.

It is remarkable that all patients with glossitis mediana rhombica were over 30 years of age. This suggests that (*i*) either they were unaware of their

Table 28

Age and sex distribution of patients with glossitis mediana rhombica

Age (years)	Men	Women	Totals
30–39	3	1	4
40–49	2	—	2
50–59	4	2	6
Totals	9	3	12

condition for some time, or that (*ii*) suspicions concerning the etiological role of infection (probably fungal) rather than congenital abnormality are justified. Of our 12 patients 11 were in fact unaware of their lesion, and one patient had known of it for 10 years. Five patients had no symptoms whatsoever, but two complained of sensitivity of the tongue, mostly to hot or sour foods.

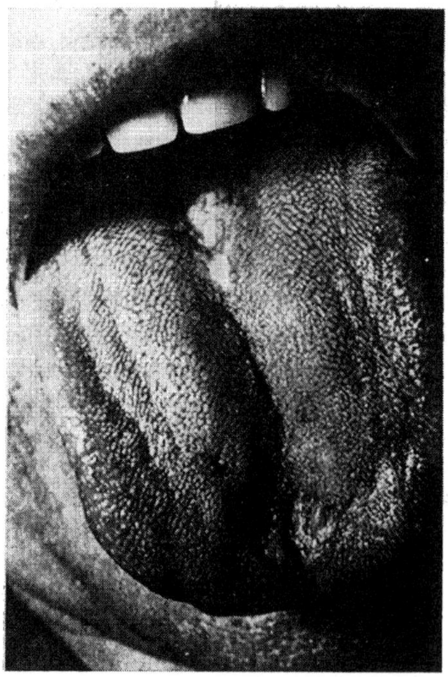

Fig. 20. Verrucous leukoplakia developed in a 50-year-old female patient at the site of median rhomboid glossitis. The lesion improved temporarily on antimycotic treatment

As to possible etiological factors, eight patients were smokers, and from two positive isolations of Candida albicans were made. Six of the seven patients wore a prosthesis, which may have predisposed them to fungal infection.

Development of leukoplakia in the area of the glossitis mediana rhombica occurred in two cases (Fig. 20 and see also Fig. 40). Of the 12 patients, nine were available for follow-up study over periods from 2 to 12 years (average 5.2 years). The methods and results of treatment of the cases available for re-examination are shown in Table 29. Some patients were treated with several methods.

Complete healing of the lesion occurred in four cases after either total excision, reduction or cessation of smoking, or antimycotic treatment. All four healed lesions were of the smooth-surfaced type (see colour photo 7 and Fig. 42). The two protuberant verrucous lesions were recurrent despite surgical excision and subsequent antimycotic therapy (see Fig. 19). The remaining five patients reported that their tongue lesion had either improved markedly, or nearly disappeared after periodic treatment with Nystatin, only to reappear after withdrawal of the fungicide. In no case was the lesion aggravated by treatment. Carcinomatous change was not observed.

Histological examination was performed in four cases. Our findings corresponded with those of other investigators (Cooke 1962, Pinkert 1967, Seifert and Vossmeyer 1978). Rete pegs were elongated and inflammatory changes were found in the subepithelial connective tissue (Fig. 21). In a single case,

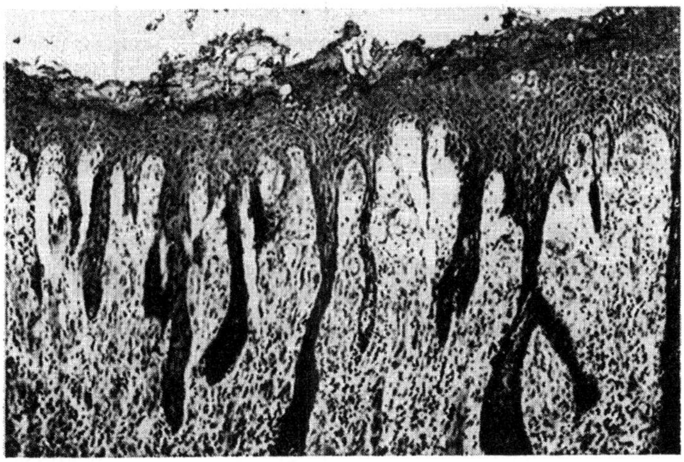

Fig. 21. Microscopic appearance of median rhomboid glossitis. The atrophic epithelium extends finger-like rete pegs deeply into the connective tissue. The surface of the lesion is parakeratotic. Marked inflammatory cell reaction in the connective tissue

Table 29

Methods and results of treatment

Method of treatment	Healed	Improved	Unchanged	Worse	Totals
Reduction of smoking	1	1	—	—	2
Antimycotic agent	1	8	—	—	9
Vitamin(s)	—	—	1	—	1
Surgical excision	2	2	—	—	4
Totals	4	11	1	—	16*

* In some cases several methods of treatment were employed.

in which glossitis mediana rhombica was associated with leukoplakia, a moderate epithelial dysplasia was also present (see Fig. 41).

To summarize our opinions on the possible etiological rôle of certain lingual lesions in oral leukoplakia or in concomitant malignant change, it appears that atrophic conditions that result from inflammation of mucosa may predispose to hyperkeratosis and cracking and thereby to malignant change. Although patients with glossitis migrans had no leukoplakia despite localized atrophy of the lingual mucosa, glossitis rhombica and, especially, the "mirror tongue" lesion accompanied by anaemia seemed to be associated with the development of oral leukoplakia or carcinoma. It follows that patients with the latter two lesions require careful observation, elimination of irritating factors and treatment for the basic disorder, to prevent progression to a precancerous or carcinomatous state.

As to the importance of the *etiological factors* considered, the following conclusions have been drawn from our own experience and from observations of other authors:

Smoking habit: 83% of patients with leukoplakia and 77% of those in whom cancer developed from leukoplakia were habitual smokers. Histological examination revealed no notable difference between the incidence of epithelial dysplasia in smokers and non-smokers with leukoplakia. This and the related observations of Einhorn and Wersäll (1967) and Roed-Petersen (1971) may support the conclusion that while an etiological or at least predisposing role of smoking is highly likely in oral leukoplakia, evidence is lacking for a similar role in malignant transformation (Cawson 1975).

The greater incidence (45%) of mechanical irritating factors in the carcinoma group compared with single leukoplakia (31.9%) suggests that chronic irritation may play a role in malignant transformation.

Alcoholism and syphilis seem to have an adverse influence only in association with other causal factors; it has recently been doubted that either of them can alone account for leukoplakia or its malignant change (Anastassov and Chpatov 1967). The same argument may be applied to the influence of electrical potential differences.

The frequency of candidiasis in patients with leukoplakia (13.5%) was within the range found by other authors: Roed-Petersen et al. (1970) reported an incidence of 31%, Renstrup (1970) 23%, Daftary et al. (1972) 6.8%, and Burkhardt and Seifert (1977) 13%. Differences in the percentage occurrence of candidiasis in oral leukoplakia can be attributed to dissimilarities in methodology and to geographical conditions. The high portion (61%) of candidiasis in our erosive leukoplakias indicates the important role of this infection in the development of this clinical type (Jepsen and Winther 1965, Nater et al. 1977). Renstrup (1970) observed a similarly high incidence (65%) of candidiasis in her patients with "speckled" leukoplakia. It should be noted that in many cases, candidiasis has been associated with dysplasia of oral epithelium (Roed-Petersen et al. 1970, Burkhardt and Seifert 1977).

Among the inflammatory and atrophic conditions of the oral mucosa, glossitis mediana rhombica and the 'mirror tongue' of anaemia seem to promote the development of leukoplakia and ultimately of carcinoma. This indicates the indirect involvement of endogenous factors in the progression through a precancerous to a cancerous state.

Finally mention should briefly be made of investigations into the possible influence of immune mechanisms on the development and malignant transformation of leukoplakia. Roed-Petersen et al. (1973) demonstrated cell-mediated hypersensitivity, and Lehner et al. (1973) cell-mediated immune definiency in patients with leukoplakia by use of the leukocyte migration test. Lehner (1971), Burkhardt and Seifert (1977) as well as Löning et al. (1977) observed by immuno-histological studies a correlation between cellular immunological competence and the incidence of dysplasia and/or carcinoma. The last cited authors observed that in cases with dysplasia and carcinoma, the percentage immunoglobulin (IgA, IgG) content of plasma cells was twice as high as in simple leukoplakia without dysplasia. Dabelsteen (1980) demonstrated the loss of epithelial blood group antigens "A" and "B" in oral premalignant lesions. Shillitoe and Silverman (1979) and Shillitoe (1980) found a relationship between Herpes simplex virus 1 antibodies and malignization of leukoplakia. The importance of these factors in the malignant transformation of leukoplakias is being investigated in continuing experiments.

CHAPTER III

TRANSFORMATIONS IN THE CLINICAL TYPE OF LEUKOPLAKIA DURING LONGITUDINAL STUDIES

Our previous longitudinal studies (Bánóczy and L. Sugár 1972) revealed cancer development in 28% of erosive leukoplakias. Roed-Petersen (1971) observed carcinoma in 9.1% of the 331 "speckled" leukoplakias in his longitudinal study. In other clinical types of leukoplakia, the frequency of malignant transformation was only 1.8% among our patients, and 1.3% among those of Roed-Petersen (1971).

No information, however, emerged from these studies whether "erosive" or "speckled" leukoplakia, which satisfies the criteria of a precan- cerous lesion, represents a clinically and pathologically discrete disease, or simply an advanced variant of either simple or verrucous leukoplakia. It remained to be clarified whether the various clinical types of oral leukoplakia were different stages of the same lesion, or each representative of an independent entity (Bánóczy and L. Sugár 1975, L. Sugár and Bánóczy 1975).

We examined the frequency of type to type transitions, and the impact of different factors on these. "Improved" and "spread" cases (Bánóczy and L. Sugár 1972) in the large group available for longitudinal study–and hence under continuous medical supervision–were examined for the frequency of changes in clinical type. "Improvement" was understood to be either a decrease in the size of the lesion or a transformation from a severe (erosive) to a milder (simple or verrucous) type, while, conversely, "spread" meant the lesion's expansion, or a change from mild to severe type, e.g. simplex to erosive.

A change of type was observed in 66 (12.7%) of the 520 oral leukoplakias in our study (Table 30).

The change was toward improvement in 47 cases (9%). Of these cases, which all moved into "simplex" category, 40 had originally been erosive, and seven had been verrucous. Among the 19 (3.7%) cases classified as "spread", six transformed from simple to verrucous, while the remaining 13 cases were respectively simple to erosive and verrucous to erosive transformations. Therefore *in the course of longitudinal studies distinct transformations in the clinical type of leukoplakia could be observed.*

Analysis of the various categories of leukoplakia for the frequency of transformation of type showed that among the 265 simple, 173 verrucous

Table 30

Distribution of regressive and progressive changes in the clinical types of leukoplakia

Type of leukoplakia \ Nature of change	Improved cases			Spread		
	Reduction in size	Type change	Total	Increase in size	Progressive type change	Total
Simplex	41	47	88	8	—	4
Verrucous	32	—	32	15	6	21
Erosive	11	—	11	9	13	22
Totals	84	47	131	28	19	47

and 82 erosive leukoplakias 16 (6 %), 10 (5.7 %) and 40 (48.7 %), respectively, changed to another type. It follows that *erosive leukoplakia proved to be the most changeable among the three clinical types.* The site distribution of the leukoplakias subject to type transformation is shown in Table 31.

The lesions showing "improvement" (v. supra), were located in the commissure, buccal mucosa and lip in 30, 10 and seven cases, respectively. Lesions showing "spread" (v. supra), were found in the same sites and, additionally, in two cases each on the tongue and floor of the mouth.

A type change occurred most frequently (37.5 %) in leukoplakias of the lip, next, in nearly equal proportions (20.5 % and 20.7 %) in commissural and buccal lesions, and least often in those located on the tongue (7.4 %) and floor of the mouth (9.1 %). No type transformation occurred in lesions of the hard or soft palate, and alveolar ridge.

Table 31

Sites of leukoplakias exhibiting type transformation

Localization	Regressive lesions	Progressive lesions	Total No. of		Type change %
			Lesion showing type change	Leukoplakia	
Commissures	30	4	34	166	20.3
Buccal mucosa	10	8	18	87	20.7
Lip	7	3	10	28	35.7
Tongue	—	2	2	27	7.4
Floor of the mouth	—	2	2	22	9.1
Other	—	—	—	190	0.0
Totals	47	19	66	520	12.7

Table 32

Percentage occurrence of different etiological factors in leukoplakias showing a regressive or progressive change, and in the total groups with leukoplakia and carcinoma

Etiological factors \ Groups of patients	Regressive change	Progressive change	Total groups with leukoplakia*	Total groups with carcinoma*
Smoking habit	89.0	95.0	83.0	77.0
Mechanical irritation	42.0	42.0	31.0	45.0
Alcoholism	6.4	10.5	13.0	33.0
Electric potential difference	2.1	0.0	3.0	19.3
Candidiasis	38.0	53.0	13.5	65.0
No etiological factor	0.0	0.0	4.2	3.2
Several etiological factors	64.0	84.0	37.5	52.0

* (Bánóczy and Sugár 1972)

The distribution of etiological factors is shown in Table 32.

The proportion of patients with a smoking habit and with candidiasis was considerably higher in the group that showed changes of type than in the total groups of leukoplakia and carcinoma patients. Multifactorial etiology was also more frequent among the cases classified as "improved" and "spread" than in the total groups. Clinical observation has indicated that each type of leukoplakia may transform to another. Longitudinal studies have shown that progressive transformation from a clinically milder type to the severe erosive type occurred in 3.7 %, of the cases, while a regressive transformation from severe to milder type, i.e. an improvement, in 9.0 %.

The frequency of malignant transformation in leukoplakia (5.9 %) was greater than that of progressive cases ("spread" type) (3.7 %). This, and the large number of regressive, "improved" cases can be attributed to the regular treatment of the patients. We believe that without treatment, the proportion of progressive changes would have been higher. The time factor also seemed to be important; the mean latent period of type change was longer than the mean time period required for cancer development from leukoplakia.

In our experience the clinical types of leukoplakia regarded as less hazardous tend to transform slowly into the erosive type, which is more liable to malignant change than simple or verrucous leukoplakia. Carcinoma arises most frequently from erosive leukoplakia (Bánóczy and L. Sugár 1972, L. Sugár and Bánóczy 1970*a*, *b*), but it cannot be ruled out that simple leukoplakia may also be precancerous through progression to the erosive type. In view of this it may be stated that leukoplakia is not essentially a static lesion but one which can undergo dynamic change through different forms which require different times for malignant transformation.

As to a correlation between type change and site, 94% of the lesions showing such change were found in regions lined by a loosely bound mucous membrane, i.e. at the commissures, buccal lesions 35.7% changed their type after a time. This is in accord with the observations of Mehta and Pindborg (1974) that spontaneous regression was most frequent in leukoplakia of the upper lip, commissures and buccal mucosa. It follows that lesions of non-keratinized oral epithelium are more liable than those of keratinized epithelium to both regressive and progressive change. Hyperkeratotic fusions of normally keratinized epithelium also seemed to be more stable to judge from the absence of type transformations in lesions of the palate or alveolar ridge. Against this the leukoplakias of the tongue and floor of the mouth showed exclusively progressive changes ("spread"), despite the fact that principles and methods of treatment were the same in every case. The type changes in our group of oral leukoplakias were too few to permit definitive conclusions, but we substantiated our earlier observations that lesions of the tongue and floor of the mouth are more liable to malignant change than those occurring in other sites (Bánóczy and L. Sugár 1972).

Analysis of the distribution of etiological factors suggested that smoking and candidiasis largely influenced type change. Among the 47 patients showing regression 28 had stopped smoking completely. Against this Mehta and Pindborg (1974), and Mehta et al. (1972) concluded from 5-year and 10-year follow-up studies of Indian patients that some leukoplakia in smokers regressed even when the habit was not given up. Gupta et al. (1980) observed spontaneous regression annually in 4–8% of their leukoplakia patients.

In our experience, stopping the smoking habit has a beneficial influence chiefly on the verrucous and erosive types of leukoplakia. The high incidence of candidiasis may account for the great frequency of erosive leukoplakias among the cases showing type transformation; Renstrup (1970) and ourselves found candidiasis in 61 and 65%, respectively, of cases with speckled or erosive leukoplakia. We frequently observed transformation of a milder type of leukoplakia to an erosive lesion in those cases where candidiasis supervened because of a predisposing factor such as use of a prosthesis. Antimycotic therapy in such cases was often followed by regression to a milder type. This observation points to the importance of definitive treatment.

The disposition to transformation in erosive leukoplakias could equally account for both their predisposition to malignant change and their greater responsiveness to treatment compared to milder types. It follows that *continuous medical care and appropriate treatment can prevent* not only the malignant transformation of erosive leukoplakia, but also *the progression of the clinical types regarded as mild to the potentially malignant, unstable erosive type.*

CHAPTER IV

COMPARATIVE STUDY OF THE CLINICAL TYPES AND HISTOLOGICAL CHARACTERISTICS OF ORAL LEUKOPLAKIA

The interrelationships between the clinical and histological forms of oral leukoplakia have been little studied. During the last twenty or so years, Renstrup (1958) reported the histological evaluation of 80 cases, Fasske et al. (1958) of 103 cases, Luzardo-Baptista (1968) of 50 cases, Silverman and Rozen (1968) of 117 cases, Gigliardi et al. (1966) of 221 cases, Shafer and Waldron (1961) of 332 cases and Waldron and Shafer (1975) of 3,256 cases identified clinically as oral leukoplakia. Their evaluation was based on determination of the frequency of occurrence of hyperkeratosis, parakeratosis, acanthosis, hyperplasia, atrophy, dysplasia and carcinoma. They generally concluded that the lesions known collectively as leukoplakia in the clinical sense could not be regarded as precancerous unless firm histological evidence of premalignancy was available. Similar considerations prompted J. Sugár (1961, 1968) as well as Venkei and J. Sugár (1965) to classify the precancerous lesions into three histomorphological categories, (*i*) diffuse epithelial hyperplasia, (*ii*) focal epithelial proliferation and/or atypia, and (*iii*) severe atypia, incipient carcinoma. Burkhardt and Seifert (1977) also determined the percentage occurrences of dysplasia and carcinoma in situ in their histological analysis of 656 oral leukoplakias. It should be noted that, on the other hand, histologically verified invasive or carcinoma in situ would not infrequently appear clinically as an oral leukoplakia (Shafer 1975, Kuffer and Fiore-Donno 1977).

Recent histological studies have been concerned with the quantitative determination of certain microscopic characteristics of oral leukoplakia, and with the diagnostic differentiation of leukoplakia from keratosis and lichen planus on this basis (Kramer et al. 1970*a*, *b*). The main histological characteristics of leukoplakia were identified by computer analysis, with special regard to those prevalent in leukoplakias subject to malignant transformation (Kramer 1969, El-Labban et al. 1971, Kramer et al. 1974). In Hungarian studies, the prevalence of certain histological characteristics within the given clinical types was assessed by retrospective analysis of biopsies obtained in 130 cases. Sonkodi and Győri (1975) found that of the pathological keratinization patterns, hyperkeratosis was most frequent in categories in which signs of malignant transformation were also present.

The above-cited authors based their histological examinations on leukoplakia in general, while Pindborg et al. (1963) pursued the epithelial changes occurring in the "speckled" (precancerous) type of leukoplakia in particular. In my previous investigations into possible correlations between clinical types and keratinization patterns of 134 oral leukoplakias (Bánóczy 1968) I found orthokeratosis in 60 and 57 % of the simple and verrucous leukoplakia cases, respectively, but parakeratosis in the greater part (57 %) of the erosive leukoplakias. Parakeratosis was associated with epithelial hyperplasia in 86 % of the cases, while orthokeratosis in only 42 %. According to the available literature, this particular aspect of the interrelationship between the clinical and histological types of leukoplakia has not been studied.

To obtain more information on the problem, further studies were carried out to identify the major histological changes that can be related to clinical type, and the characteristics of the cases showing epithelial dysplasia.

For light microscopic examination either a punch biopsy was taken with a 4 mm or 5 mm corneal trephine, or the lesion was excised *in toto* with a scalpel. Both procedures were performed under local anaesthesia with 2 % Lidocaine. The specimens were fixed in 10 % formalin, embedded in paraffin, and the sections cut were stained with haematoxylin and eosin.

Sections obtained from 500 clinical cases of oral leukoplakia were examined and evaluated for the following changes (Bánóczy and Csiba 1970, 1972, Bánóczy et al. 1979).

EPITHELIAL CHANGES

Orthokeratosis: a normal state, where cells of the superficial layers of epithelium are nearly homogeneous, eosinophilic and anuclear, with a stratum granulosum always present (Fig. 22).

Hyperorthokeratosis: a pathological state characterized by increased thickness of the orthokeratotic layer exceeding the normal for that region (Fig. 22).

Parakeratosis: the superficial epithelial cells are flat and acidophilic, with pyknotic nuclei; a stratum granulosum may or may not be present (Fig. 23).

Hyperparakeratosis: a pathological alteration characterized by increased thickness of the parakeratotic layer exceeding the normal for that area (Fig. 24).

Dyskeratosis: a pathological alteration characterized by keratinization of single cells or groups of cell in the stratum spinosum (Fig. 25).

Hyperplasia: proliferation of cells in all epithelial layers, accounting for an increase of thickness (see Fig. 23).

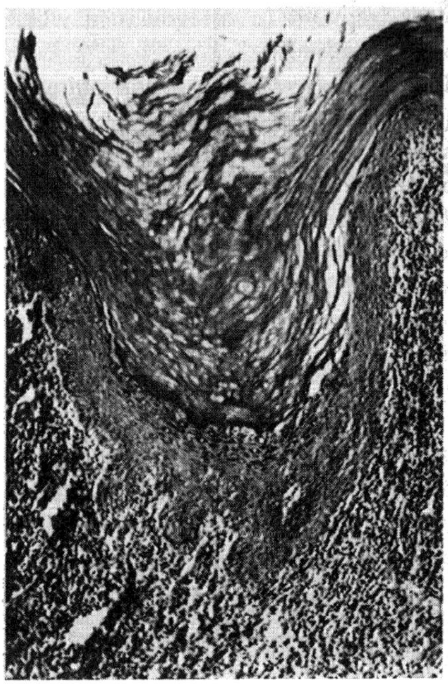

Fig. 22. Microscopic appearance of orthokeratosis (*a*) and hyperorthokeratosis (*b*). The topmost layers of the epithelium are almost homogeneous, eosinophilic and anucletaed. There is a distinct stratum granulosum. The connective tissue contains inflammatory cells. H. & E., × 125

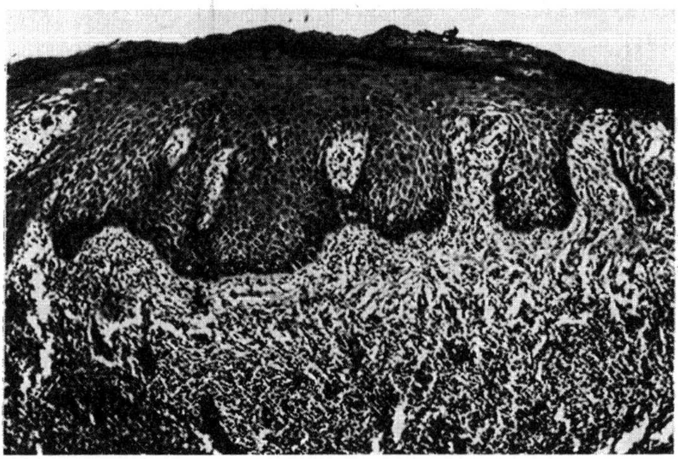

Fig. 23. Microscopic appearance of epithelial hyperplasia and parakeratosis. Note quantitative increase of cell elements in all layers of the epithelium, with acanthosis and basal-cell hyperplasia. The superficial cell rows are flat, with pyknotic nuclei. The connective tissue is infiltrated by inflammatory cells. H. & E., ×125

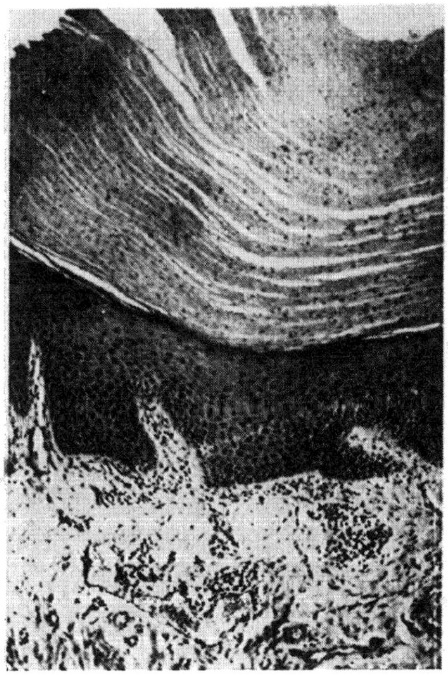

Fig. 24. Microscopic appearance of hyperparakeratosis: the thickness of the parakeratotic layer is increased over normal. H. & E., ×125

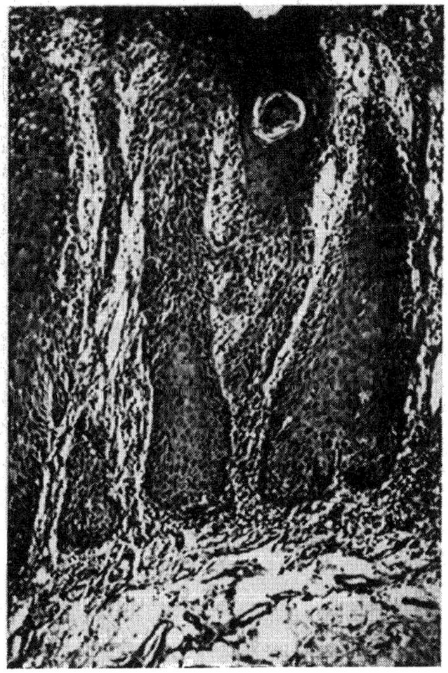

Fig. 25. Microscopic appearance of dyskeratosis. Note aggregation of keratinized cells in the spinous layer. H. & E., ×125

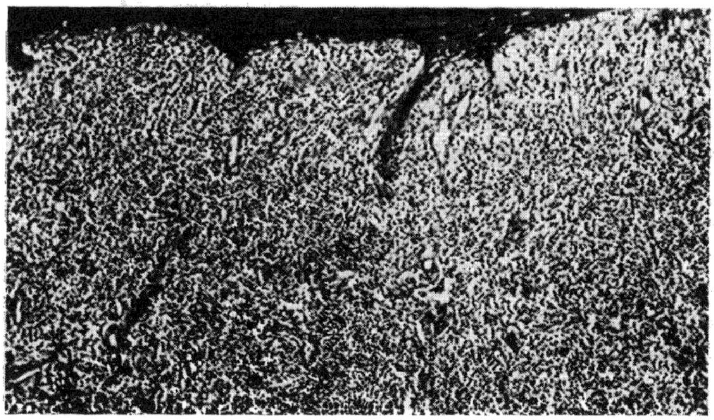

Fig. 26. Microscopic appearance of epithelial atrophy. Quantitative decrease and flattening of the epithelial cells lead to a reduction in epithelial thickness. The connective tissue is infiltrated by inflammatory cells. H. & E., ×125

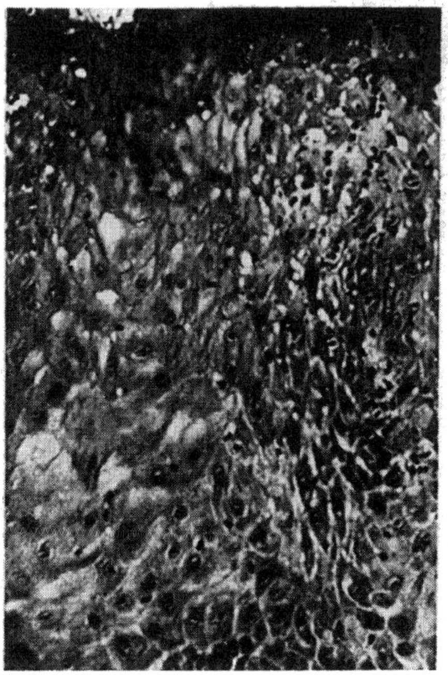

Fig. 27. Microscopic appearance of intracellular oedema (hydropic degeneration). The cells are swollen and round, with a honeycomb-like cytoplasm, but preserved nuclear staining. H. & E., ×250

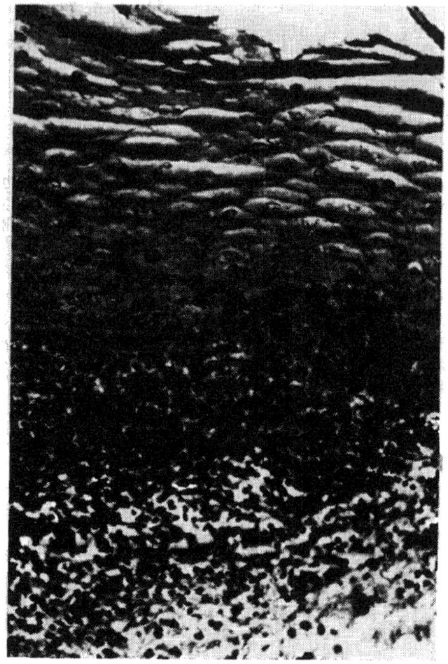

Fig. 28. Microscopic appearance of intercellular oedema (spongiosis). The intercellular spaces are dilated, and the tight junctions are open. H. & E., ×250

Acanthosis: an increase in the number of cells of the stratum spinosum. Basal-cell hyperplasia: an increase in the number of cells in the basal layer of epithelium (see Fig. 23 and 31).

Atrophy: reduction of the normal thickness of epithelium due to a decrease in the number of its cells (Fig. 26).

Intra-epithelial oedema: (*a*) intracellular oedema (hydropic degeneration): swollen, rounded epithelial cells with a honeycomb-like cytoplasm but preserved staining affinity of the nucleus (Fig. 27). (*b*) Intercellular oedema (spongiosis): dilatation of the intercellular spaces and disruption of the intercellular junctions due to the accumulation of fluid between the epithelial cells (Fig. 28).

Vacuolar degeneration: the cytoplasmic structure is indistinct, and the nucleus is pushed to the cell periphery. Vacuolar degeneration may occur in the

Fig. 29. Microscopic appearance of vacuolar degeneration. Note loss of definition of cytoplasmic structure and displacement of the nuclei towards the cell periphery. Dysplasia is indicated by an increased nuclear : cytoplasmic ratio, nuclear polymorphism and nuclear hyperchromatism. H. & E., ×250

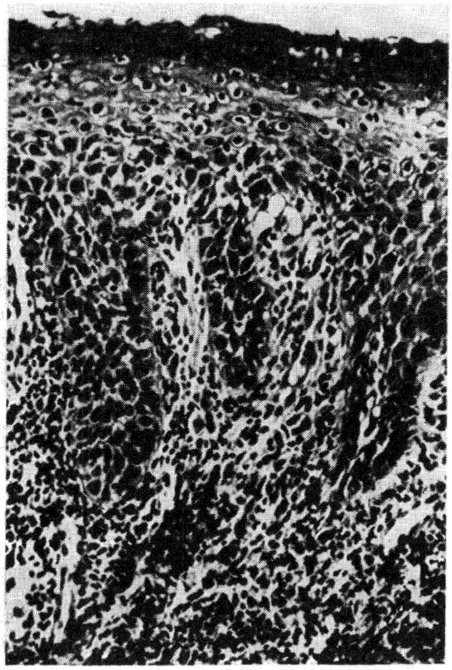

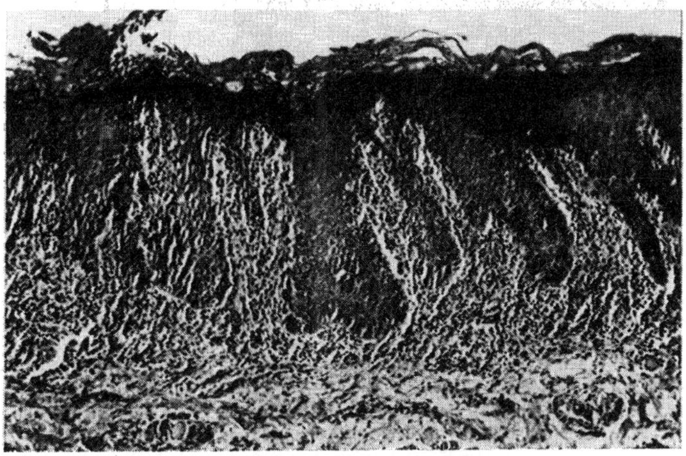

Fig. 30. Microscopic appearance of dysplasia. Note irregular stratification of epithelium, with drop-like rete pegs, and inflammatory cell infiltration in the connective tissue. H. & E., ×125

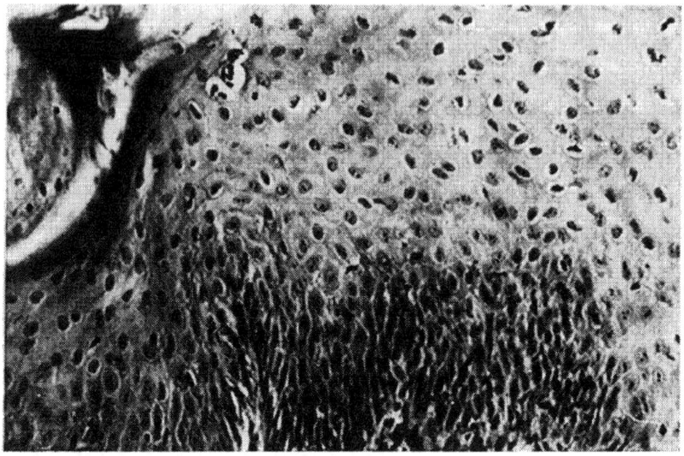

Fig. 31. Basal-cell hyperplasia. H. & E., ×250

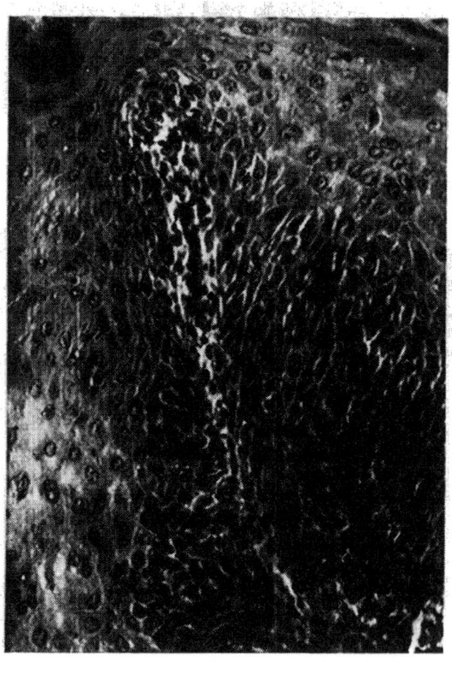

Fig. 32. Epithelial dysplasia. Note quantitative increase of mitotic cells, abnormal mitoses, nuclear hypertrophy and hyperchromatism, and increased numbers of nucleoli per cell. H. & E., ×250

stratum spinosum or stratum germinativum. This change may be called "liquefaction degeneration" but El-Labban and Kramer (1975) have questioned its correctness on the basis of electron microscopic observations, while

Fig. 33. Altered polarity of basal cells. H. & E., ×250

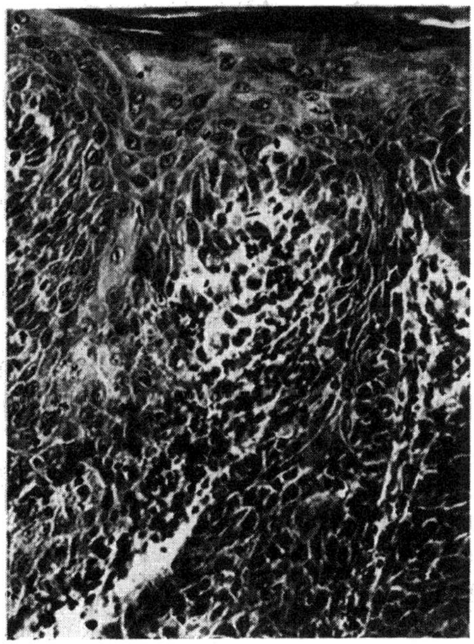

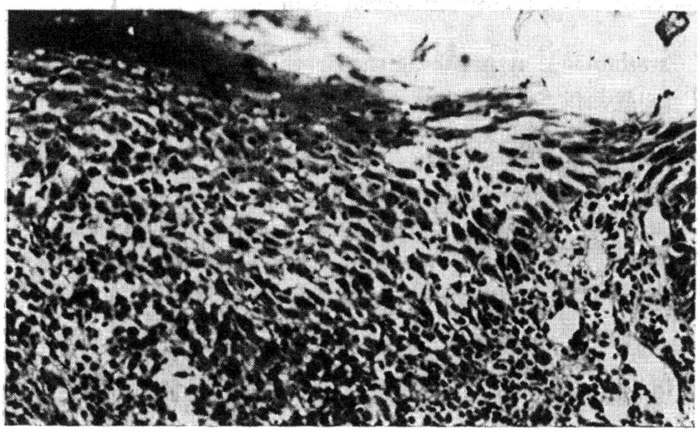

Fig. 34. Splitting of intercellular junctions in all layers of the epithelium. H. & E., ×250

failing to propose another name. This change may cause separation of the epithelium from the subepithelial connective tissue by the deposition of fluid (subepithelial bulla formation) (Fig. 29).

Dysplasia: a collective term for all disorders of epithelial cell differentiation except invasive and carcinoma in situ. The histological diagnosis of dysplasia was established if two or more of the following signs were present together:

1. abnormal stratification of the epithelium (Fig. 30)
2. basal-cell hyperplasia (Fig. 31)
3. drop-shaped rete pegs (Fig. 30)
4. increase of mitotic activity (with few abnormal mitoses) (Fig. 32)
5. altered polarity of basal cells (Fig. 33)
6. increase of the nuclear cytoplasmic ratio (Fig. 29)
7. nuclear polymorphism (Fig. 29)
8. nuclear and nucleolar hyperchromatism (Figs 29 and 32)
9. increase of nucleolar size (Fig. 32)
10. keratinization of single cells or groups of cell in the stratum spinosum (Fig. 25)
11. loss of intercellular junctions (Fig. 34)

Epithelial dysplasia was graded as mild, moderately severe or severe depending on the presence of either two, two to four, or five or more of the above signs.

CONNECTIVE TISSUE CHANGES

Inflammation: a pathological condition characterized by the presence of dispersed or aggregated chronic inflammatory cells in the subepithelial connective tissue (see Figs 22, 23, 26 and 30).

Hyaline degeneration: a pathological condition characterized by replacement of degenerated elastic fibres by a hyaline fibrous tissue (Fig. 35).

The above histological criteria were also used for the diagnostic differentiation of 67 cases of lichen planus, leukoedema exfoliativum mucosae oris and morsicatio buccarum et labiorum from leukoplakia (see below).

COMPARATIVE ANALYSIS OF NON-DYSPLASTIC CASES

Of the 500 cases diagnosed clinically as leukoplakia, 48 (9.6%), 120 (24%) and 332 (66.4%) were identified histologically as carcinoma, epithelial dysplasia and non-dysplastic simple hyperplasia or hyperkeratosis of epithelium, respectively. The histologically verified cases of carcinoma are outside the scope of this study, and the cases of epithelial dysplasia are analyzed separately in the second part of this chapter.

The distribution of the main histological changes between the various clinical types of lesion in the 332 non-malignant, non-dysplastic cases is

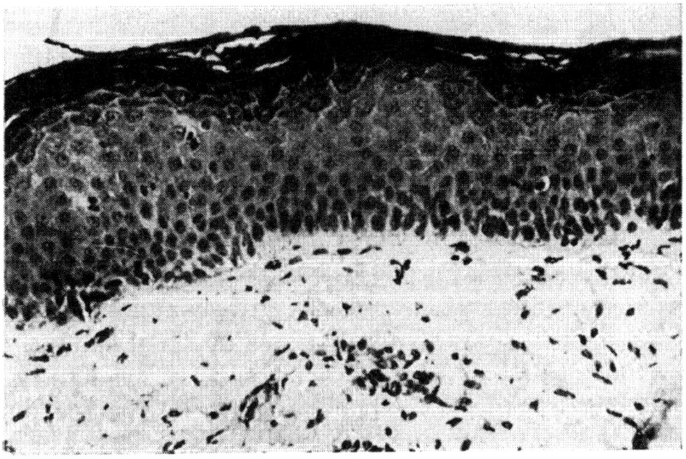

Fig. 35. Hyaline degeneration. The degenerated elastic fibres are replaced by fibrous hyaline tissue. H. & E., ×250

shown in Table 33. In this particular group 173, 103 and 56 patients, respectively, had simple, verrucous and erosive leukoplakia.

Histologically simple leukoplakia was characterized by hyperkeratosis, the presence of a stratum granulosum and by hyperplasia, while in verrucous leukoplakia there was in addition to these changes a marked dyskeratosis, and inflammation of the subepithelial connective tissue. In erosive leukoplakia para-

Table 33

Numerical and percentage distribution of histopathological alterations among the different clinical types in 332 cases of oral leukoplakia (several changes were simultaneously present in most cases)

Type of histological change	Clinical types of oral leukoplakia						Total	
	Simplex		Verrucous		Erosive			
	No.	%	No.	%	No.	%	No.	%
Hyperorthokeratosis	79	45.7	73	70.9	32	57.1	184	55.4
Parakeratosis	15	10.4	13	12.6	14	25.0	42	12.7
Hyperparakeratosis	28	16.2	35	34.0	35	62.5	98	29.5
Stratum granulosum	44	25.4	47	45.6	17	30.4	108	32.5
Dyskeratosis	10	5.8	23	22.3	25	44.6	58	17.5
Intra-epithelial oedema	37	21.4	31	30.1	15	26.8	83	25.0
Hyperplasia	60	34.7	75	72.8	50	89.3	185	55.7
Atrophy	33	19.1	30	29.1	14	25.0	77	23.2
Connective tissue inflammation	54	31.2	77	74.8	48	85.7	179	53.9
Hyaline degeneration	15	8.7	11	10.7	9	16.1	35	10.5

keratosis, hyperparakeratosis, dyskeratosis, epithelial hyperplasia and epithelial connective tissue inflammation were characteristically present.

Certain histological changes were variously present in the different histological types of leukoplakia. The variations had a high statistical significance in respect of connective tissue inflammation, hyperplasia, dyskeratosis, hyperparakeratosis and hyperorthokeratosis ($p < 0.01$).

Our studies were concerned with the detection of any correlation between clinical type and histological characteristics, to ascertain whether or not the clinical appearance of oral leukoplakia was indicative of its severity. In a similar study covering the histological analysis of 656 leukoplakia cases, Burkhardt and Seifert (1977) demonstrated a relationship between clinical type and progressive, microscopic changes. They found that the microscopic appearance of leukoplakia simplex was usually simple epithelial hyperplasia, while verrucous and erosive leukoplakia showed, as a rule, a papilliferous endophytic or exophytic proliferation, in frequent association with dysplasia. In our simplex and verrucous leukoplakias we usually saw hyperorthokeratosis, a stratum granulosum, dyskeratosis, and slight inflammation of the subepithelial connective tissue. Similar microscopic alterations have been observed in one subtype of leukoplakia simplex, a circumscribed, white patch without inflammatory involvement of the mucosa (Klein-Szántó et al. 1976, Bánóczy et al. 1977, Schroeder et al. 1978). In contrast para- and hyperkeratosis were prevalent in erosive leukoplakia, together with hyperplasia, dyskeratosis, and connective tissue inflammation. Those are the histological characteristics described by Pindborg et al. (1963) in the clinical type which they described as "speckled" (and we call "erosive"). Shafer and Waldron (1961) suggested that greyish-white and red, granular lesions of this type not infrequently harbour a carcinoma in situ. L. Sugár and Bánóczy (1970*a*, *b*) observed that cancer most frequently developed from the erosive type, and Pindborg et al. (1963), Shafer and Waldron (1961), as well as Silverman and Rozen (1968) reported the same for the speckled type; these clinical observations are in accordance with the histological evidence. Several authors (Cahn et al. 1961, Turesky et al. 1961, Shafer and Waldron 1961) have reported the frequent association of parakeratosis with epithelial hyperplasia. Renstrup and Main (1966) concluded that the high mitotic index found in association with parakeratosis indicated an increased tendency to proliferation. Cahn and co-workers (1961), and Renstrup (1958) observed an increased frequency of atypia and of the development of carcinoma in situ in parakeratotic leukoplakias. Kovács (1962*b*), too, found a greater malignant transformation rate in the presence of parakeratosis. Both us and Pindborg et al. (1963) found a superficial parakeratosis in practically all carcinomas developing from leukoplakia, including the three types of carcinoma in situ referred to in this report.

Of course, it cannot be ruled out that cancer may occasionally develop from leukoplakia simplex, or at least be already present at the microscopic level (Bakács 1962). This observation does not, however, interfere in any way with the conclusion which emerges from the present study. This is that the clinically most advanced (erosive) form of oral leukoplakia which is generally regarded as a precancerosis usually exhibit more severe—pre-malignant—changes at the histological level than the other forms.

The changes in subepithelial connective tissue associated with leukoplakia have been little studied. Cooke (1956), Pinkus et al. (1963), as well as Smith and Renstrup (1970) hold the view that the origin of the inflammatory cell reaction is unclear, and unrelated to the lesion. In contrast, Lehner (1971) and Burkhardt and Seifert (1977) found a correlation between the presence of potentially immunocompetent cells (immunoblasts and plasma cells) and the incidence of dysplasia or carcinoma.

Kramer et al. (1970*a*, *b*) observed a quantitative increase in Russell bodies in leukoplakias with epithelial dysplasia. Recently Löning et al. (1977) concluded from investigations into humoral and cell-mediated immune mechanism that 60% of non-dysplastic leukoplakias, and 100% of dysplastic leukoplakias and oral carcinomas were associated with an inflammatory reaction of the connective tissue. The proportions of the different inflammatory cell types did not differ between the two groups.

In our own experience, the incidence of connective tissue inflammation varied with the clinical type, and it increased with the tendency to malignant change. Accordingly, inflammatory change was more frequently associated with verrucous and erosive types than with simple leukoplakia.

INCIDENCE OF EPITHELIAL DYSPLASIA AND LONGITUDINAL STUDY OF LEUKOPLAKIAS WITH DYSPLASIA

In an attempt to define the histological characteristics of frankly precancerous lesions within the group of leukoplakia, the cases with a histological evidence of dysplasia were segregated for special analysis on the presumption of their greater liability to malignant transformation (J. Sugár 1961, 1968, Venkei and J. Sugár 1965). The incidence and outcome of dysplastic changes in oral leukoplakia have been received little attention (Mehta et al. 1969*b*, Mincer et al. 1972, Pindborg and Roed-Petersen 1973, Waldron and Shafer 1975, Burkhardt and Seifert 1977, Pindborg et al. 1977). Opinions have therefore been divergent as to the correct therapeutic approach to dysplastic leukoplakia.

We determined the incidence and severity of epithelial dysplasia in our group of leukoplakia and the frequency of dysplastic histological features in relation to clinical type, in order to evaluate its importance in longitudinal studies (Bánóczy and Csiba 1976*a*, *b*).*

Epithelial dysplasia was found in 120 (24%) of 500 cases, diagnosed clinically as leukoplakia, and covered in our histological study.

The dysplastic change was graded as mild, moderately severe and severe in 25 (20%), 72 (60%) and 23 (19.5%) cases, respectively.

The frequencies of the different histological characteristics are shown in Table 34. Irregular stratification of epithelium, drop-shaped rete pegs, and hyperplasia of the basal-cell layer were the most frequent changes (see Figs 30 and 31).

Table 35 shows the age and sex distribution of the patients in correlation with the grade of epithelial dysplasia. Of the 120 patients with epithelial dysplasia 104 (86.7%) were men and 16 (13.3%) were women.

The frequency of epithelial dysplasia tended to increase after 40 years of age, with a peak incidence (62.5%) between 50 and 69 years.

The calculated age distribution of dysplastic leukoplakias, based on age groups of the 1960 and 1970 census, is correlated in Table 36 with the actual number and percentage occurrence of such cases among the patients studied.

The uneven distribution of dysplasia in the groups above 20 years of age indicates age dependence. The incidence (relative to group size) was highest

Table 34

Percentage occurrence of certain histological characteristics in cases with epithelial dysplasia

Histological characteristics	Frequency of occurrence %
Irregular stratification of epithelium (Fig. 37)	75.0
Basal cell hyperplasia (Fig. 31)	43.3
Drop-shaped rete pegs (Fig. 37)	68.3
Increase of mitoses (Fig. 32)	2.5
Altered polarity of basal cells (Fig. 33)	23.3
Increased nuclear : cytoplasmic ratio (Fig. 37)	13.3
Nuclear polymorphism (Fig. 29)	15.0
Nuclear hyperchromatism (Fig. 37)	10.0
Nucleolar enlargement (Fig. 32)	12.5
Keratinization of single cells or groups of cells in the stratum spinosum (Fig. 25)	35.8
Loss of intercellular attachment (Fig. 37)	18.3

* Excerpted with permission from Oral Surg. Oral Med. Oral Pathol. **42**: 766–774 1976; copyrighted by The O. V. Mosby Company, St. Louis, Missouri U.S.A.

Table 35

Interrelationship of the grade of epithelial dysplasia with the patient's age and sex

Age (years) \ Grade of dysplasia	Men				Women			Totals		
	Mild	Moderately severe	Severe	Total	Mild	Moderately severe	Severe	Men	Women	%
20–29	—	1	1	2	—	—	—	—	2	1.7
30–39	1	7	2	10	—	1	1	2	12	10.0
40–49	5	7	4	16	—	3	—	3	19	15.8
50–59	6	21	8	35	1	2	1	4	39	32.5
60–69	8	19	2	29	2	3	2	7	36	30.0
>70	2	8	2	12	—	—	—	—	12	10.0
Totals	22	63	19	104	3	9	4	16	120	100.0

between 60 and 69 years, but nearly as high from 50 to 59 years. The decrease in the frequency of dysplasia from 70 years onwards was realistic in comparison to the actual size of that age group. It seems that dysplasia occurs most often between 50 and 69 years, but only half as frequently above 70 years of age.

The distribution of epithelial dysplasia in the various clinical types of leukoplakia is shown in Table 37. *Dysplasia was most frequently associated with erosive leukoplakia (46.6%), but the change was also frequent (33.0%)*

Table 36

Calculated and actual group distribution of patients with dysplastic leukoplakia (males + females)

Age (years) \ No. of cases with dysplasia	Computed No.	Actual No.	Actual / Computed
20–29	25.21	2	0.08
30–39	24.95	12	0.48
40–49	22.74	19	0.84
50–59	20.07	39	1.94
60–69	16.24	24	2.22
>70	10.79	12	1.11
Totals	120.00	120	

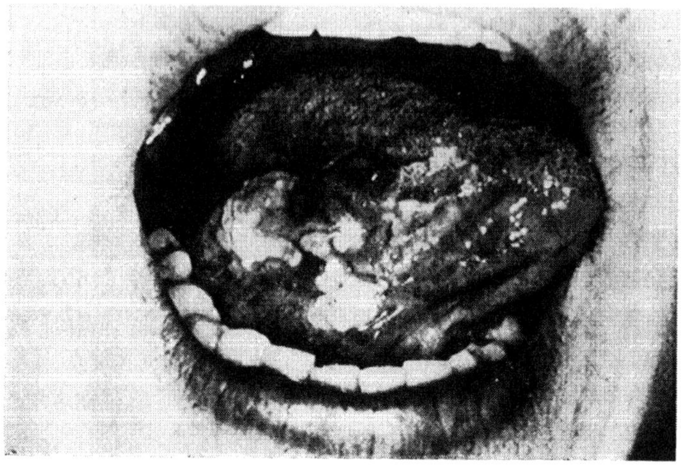

Fig. 36. Verrucous plus erosive leukoplakia on the ventral surface of the tongue of a 36-year-old, non-smoking female patient. A high electric potential difference was demonstrated between different metal restorations

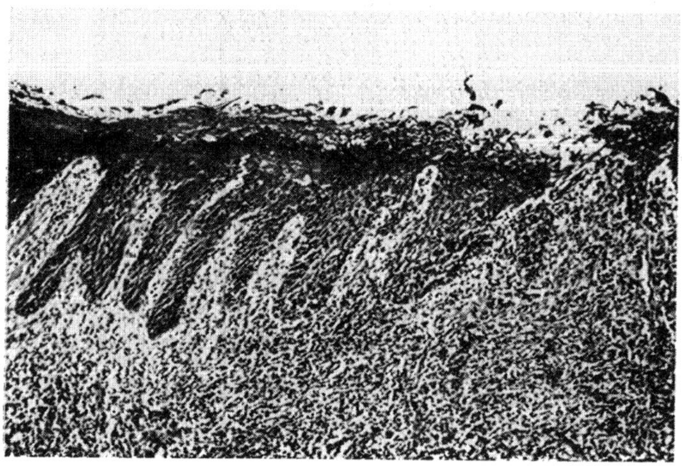

Fig. 37. Microscopic appearance of the lesion shown in Fig. 36. The epithelium exhibits superficial ulceration and hyperparakeratosis, irregular stratification with rete ridges intruding deeply into the underlying tissue, alteration of the nucleus: cytoplasmic ratio, nuclear hyperchromatism, and disruption of the intercellular junctions. The connective tissue is infiltrated by many round cells. H. & E., ×125

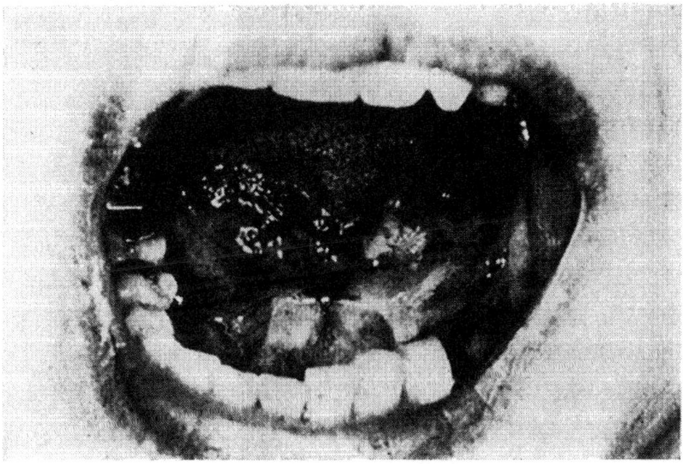

Fig. 38. Clinical appearance of the tongue shown in Fig. 36, three years later. An extensive, painless ulcer has developed at the site of the leukoplakia

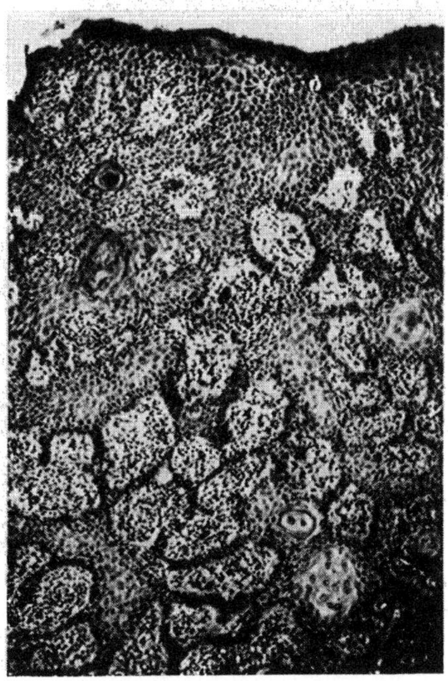

Fig. 39. Microscopic appearance of the ulceration shown in Fig. 38: squamous cell carcinoma. H. & E., ×125

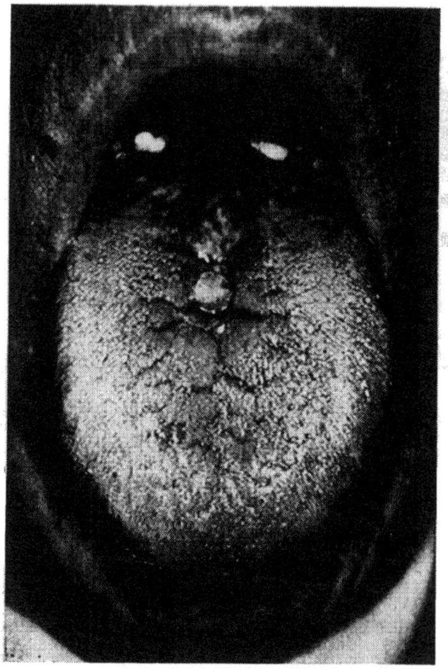

Fig. 40. Verrucous plus erosive leukoplakia in a 46-year-old male patient at the site of median rhomboid glossitis

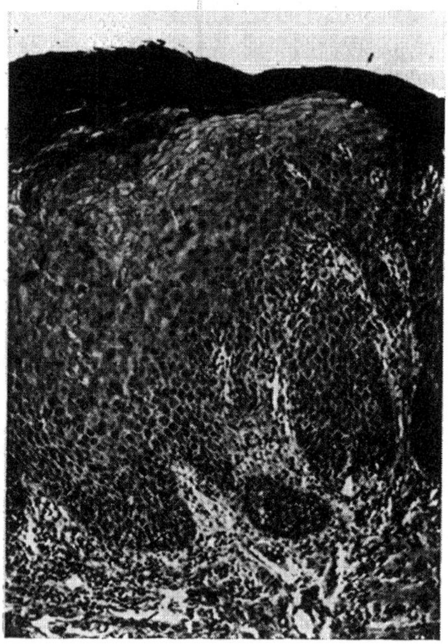

Fig. 41. Microscopic appearance of the lesion shown in Fig. 40. The thickened epithelium extends irregular finger-like ridges into the subepithelial connective tissue, which is infiltrated by inflammatory cells. H. & E., ×125

Table 37

Correlation of the grade of epithelial dysplasia with the clinical type of leukoplakia

Type of leukoplakia \ Grade of epithelial dysplasia	Mild	Moderately severe	Severe	Total	
				No.	%
Simplex	3	18	1	22	18.4
Verrucous	14	20	8	42	35.0
Erosive	8	34	14	56	46.0
Totals	25	72	23	120	100.0

in the verrucous type, while being of low incidence in the simplex type (18.4%). Statistical analysis showed its incidence to be significantly higher ($p < 0.025$) in erosive than in other forms.

Examination of the distribution of the grades of dysplasia between types showed that severe and moderately severe grades were prevalent in the erosive type, and occasional in the simplex type (Figs 36, 37, 40 and 41).

Table 38 shows the relationship of the grade of epithelial dysplasia with the site of leukoplakia. *The tongue and the lower lip were the main sites of severe dysplastic changes.*

Table 38

Correlation of the grade of epithelial dysplasia with the site of leukoplakia

Site \ Grade of epithelial dysplasia	Mild	Moderately severe	Severe	Total		Total	
				No.	%	leukoplakia group %	carcinoma* group %
Commissure	11	30	6	47	39.1	36.5	9.7
Buccal mucosa	8	16	1	25	20.8	26.3	9.7
Lip	3	13	8	24	20.0	6.5	16.1
Tongue	2	9	6	17	14.1	8.5	38.8
Hard palate	—	2	—	2	1.7	8.5	6.4
Soft palate	1	—	—	1	0.9	1.3	3.2
Floor of the mouth	—	2	—	2	1.7	5.8	9.7
Alveolar ridge	—	—	2	2	1.7	6.6	6.4
Totals	25	72	23	120	100.0	100.0	100.0

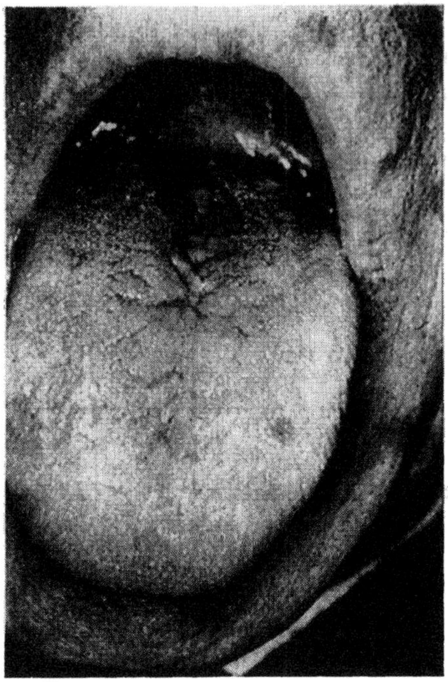

Fig. 42. Healed tongue of the patient shown in Fig. 40, eight years later. Complete healing was achieved by prohibition of smoking, antimycotic therapy, and surgical excision of the lesion

The clinical course of dysplastic leukoplakia could be followed in 68 cases for a period of 1 to 20 years, on average for 6.3 years.

Analysis of the severity of dysplasia after separating the surgically and conservatively treated cases indicated the greater efficiency of surgical treatment (Table 39). The lesions graded as moderately severe or severe did not usually recur after surgical excision (Figs 40–42).

Among the nine carcinomas (13.2% of the group with dysplasia) eight arose from leukoplakias not treated surgically. It should be noted that no regression occurred in this category (see Figs 36–39).

Examination of the further fate of dysplastic cases in relation to the site of the lesion (Table 40) showed that four of the nine carcinomas were on the tongue, while most lesions which showed healing or improvement at the commissure.

Comparison of the clinical course of the leukoplakias with the length of observation showed that healed or improved cases were more numerous within a shorter period, while after a longer time the number of unchanged, spread, and carcinomatous cases tended to increase (Table 41).

The incidence of epithelial dysplasia was higher in our group of patients with leukoplakia than in those studied by others. In India Mehta et al.

Table 39

Subsequent course of leukoplakia in relation to the grade of epithelial dysplasia and type of treatment

Grade of epithelial dysplasia / Subsequent course of leukoplakia	Treatment						Total	
	Surgical			Conservative				
	Mild	Moderately severe	Severe	Mild	Moderately severe	Severe	No.	%
Healed	9	23	4	—	—	—	36	53.0
Improved	1	6	—	1	2	—	10	14.7
Unchanged	—	—	—	1	7	2	10	14.7
Spread	—	—	1		2	—	3	4.4
Carcinoma	—	—	1	1	3	4	9	13.2
Totals	10	29	6	2	14	6	68	100.0

Table 40

Subsequent course of leukoplakia in relation to site of dysplasia

Site / Issue	Commissure	Buccal mucosa	Lip	Tongue	Palate		Floor of mouth	Alveolar ridge	Total	
					hard	soft			No.	%
Healed	22	—	9	3	2	—	—	—	36	53.0
Improved	6	2	1	—	—	1	—	—	10	14.7
Unchanged	7	1	1	1	—	—	—	—	10	14.7
Spread	1	—	—	1	—	--	1	—	3	4.4
Carcinoma	1	2	1	4	—	—	—	1	9	13.2
Totals	37	3	12	9	2	1	1	1	68	100.0

(1969*b*) found a 10.7% incidence among 723 patients with leukoplakia; later Pindborg et al. (1977) reported an incidence of 10.3%; in Denmark, Pindborg and Roed-Petersen (1973) observed dysplasia in 15.4% of 345 patients. In sections from 3,256 leukoplakias Waldron and Shafer (1975) saw slight to moderately severe dysplasia in 12.2%, and severe dysplasia and carcinoma in situ in 4.5%. In earlier studies of 184 leukoplakias, Roed-Petersen et al. (1973) found a 28.8% occurrence of epithelial dysplasia, i.e. a high incidence similar to the 24% found in the present study. The percentage occurrences given by Burkhardt and Seifert (1977) as 17%, 6% and

Table 41

Subsequent course of leukoplakia in relation to the length of the observation period

Outcome \ Observation period	>1–<2	>2–<5	>5–<10	>10–<20	Total	
					No.	%
Healed	8	14	12	2	36	36.0
Improved	1	3	3	3	10	14.7
Unchanged	—	4	4	2	10	14.7
Spread	—	—	2	1	3	4.4
Carcinoma	—	3	4	2	9	13.2
Totals	9	24	25	10	68	100.0

3%, respectively, for moderately severe dysplasia, severe dysplasia, and carcinoma in situ are, however, nearly identical with our present findings.

As to the frequency of the main histological features of epithelial dysplasia, Mehta et al. (1969*b*), and Burkhardt and Seifert (1977) found a similar frequency of basal-cell hyperplasia to ourselves. Mehta et al. (1969*b*) also observed an increase in mitotic activity and nuclear hyperchromatism, while Burkhardt and Seifert (1977) found dyskeratosis and loss of the polarity of basal cells. The latter changes were rare in our material, but irregular stratification of the epithelium and drop-shaped rete pegs were frequent.

The proportion of females among patients with dysplastic leukoplakia (13.3%) was lower than in the entire group of leukoplakias (24%). Burkhardt and Seifert (1977) found a proportion which corresponded best with percentage found (16.8%) in our previous histological series (Roed-Petersen et al. 1973). The explanation of this differences may lie in the dissimilar attitude toward biopsy in Denmark and Hungary. In Denmark biopsies were taken from all patients at the first examination, while in Hungary they were taken only from clinically dubious cases and from those not showing improvement after elimination of irritating factors. Since among the Hungarian patients women were generally more ready to co-operate with the surgeon and stop smoking than men, biopsies were required from fewer females than males. This would explain while the original proportion of 24% women fell to 16.8% by the time of histological examination. The fact that Mincer et al. (1972), and Pindborg and Roed-Petersen (1973), respectively, found 33.9 and 46.9% of females among their patients with dysplastic leukoplakia, can be attributed to the greater popularity of tobacco chewing among woman in the U.S.A. and Denmark. This is in accord with Waldron and Shafer's (1975) finding at a large proportion of females in the tobacco chewing category of patients with dysplastic leukoplakia.

The age distribution of dysplastic leukoplakia corresponds with that found in the total of leukoplakis (Bánóczy and L. Sugár 1972). Our findings differ from those of Mincer et al. (1972), as well as Pindborg and Roed-Petersen (1973) only in respect of the 30 to 39 years age group, where they observed an incidence of 3.6 and 2.0% dysplastic leukoplakia, respectively, against 10.0% in our material. A peak incidence of dysplasia was, however, most distinct among patients older than 50 years; we found it in 72.5% of them, while the above investigators, respectively found it in 83.9 and 79.6%.

Analysis of data from the dysplastic leukoplakias for the distribution of clinical type showed a dominance of erosive lesions (see Table 37). Among all erosive lesions in the total group studied, epithelial dysplasia occurred in 68% (in 56 cases out of 82). This was higher than the incidence of 51% found by Pindborg et al. (1963) among their speckled leukoplakias. The statistical significance of differences in type incidence and the increased frequency of severe dysplasia among erosive lesions (see Table 37) supports our earlier observation of a greater potential for malignant transformation in this type (Bánóczy and L. Sugár 1972), and also substantiates the earlier correlation (Bánóczy and Csiba 1972) made between the clinical type and histological structure of oral leukoplakia.

Comparison of the site distribution of dysplastic leukoplakias with that found in the total groups of leukoplakia and carcinoma (Bánóczy and L. Sugár 1972; see Table 38) revealed that while the percentage frequency of commissural and buccal sites was similar to that of the total group of leukoplakias, labial dysplasias had a site incidence similar to one found in the carcinoma group, while the frequency of the lingual site was intermediate between the two. This, and the high incidence of moderately severe to severe dysplasia in lingual and labial lesions suggests that a major risk is associated with such lesions (Seifert and Burkhardt 1979, Burkhardt 1980). This is in accord with our observation (Bánóczy and L. Sugár 1972) on a greater rate incidence of malignant change in lingual and labial leukoplakia compared to lesions in other sites, and with Waldron and Shafer's (1975) finding of a major incidence of dysplasia and carcinoma on the tongue and lip. Burkhardt and Seifert (1977) observed a similar site distribution in their patients.

In our material there were 68 patients with dysplastic leukoplakia available for longitudinal study. This group was somewhat larger than the 45, 37, and 61 patients available to Mincer et al. (1972), Pindborg and Roed-Petersen (1973), and Pindborg et al. (1977), respectively, and our observation period was also longer. We observed cancer development in 13.2% of the cases; this was close to the 11.1 % reported by Mincer et al. (1972), but considerably in excess of the incidences of 2.0 and 6.6 % found by Pindborg et al. (1977) and Pindborg and Roed-Petersen (1973). Also, the proportion of improved and healed cases, 67.7 % in our dysplastic group, was considerably higher than the 40.0 and 40.9 % reported by the latter authors. Such differences can be attributed to the fact that we treated 67 % of our cases surgically, as compared with the 44.0 % and 53 % so treated by Mincer et al. (1972), and Pindborg and Roed-Petersen (1973). Pindborg et al. (1977) also observed spontaneous regression in 14.8 % of their cases over a 7-year observation period. These and our earlier observations (L. Sugár and Bánóczy 1970*a*, *b*) have unequivocally indicated the superiority of surgical treatment over a conservative approach even in dysplastic cases.

Analysis of the progress of dysplasias at various sites has substantiated our earlier observation (Bánóczy and L. Sugár 1972) and that of Roed-Petersen (1971) that lingual leukoplakia constitutes a greater risk than lesions in other sites.

Evaluation of the outcome of dysplastic changes against time gave results which also accorded well with our earlier findings (L. Sugár and Bánóczy 1970*a*, *b*) that the malignant transformation of leukoplakia requires a distinct latent period.

CHAPTER V

CYTOLOGICAL STUDIES IN ORAL LEUKOPLAKIA

The cytological examination of oral leukoplakias has a dual purpose, it makes possible the detection of malignant change, and also gives information about the process of keratinization.

Papanicolaou and Traut's (1943) staining technique for cytological smears was first used in oral leukoplakia by Montgomery and von Haam in 1951. Since then most investigators have used the method in an attempt to detect malignant transformation, but opinions have been divergent as to its efficiency. Knychalska-Karwan (1964) found it suitable for the identification of the precise stage of the disease, and Wahi et al. (1966) differentiated between "simplex" and "active" leukoplakias by the presence or absence of atypical cells in smears. Mela (1965) distinguished five cytological classes of leukoplakia by an adaptation of Papanicolaou's gynecological cytodiagnostic method. Fasske et al. (1958, 1959*a*, *b*) and Hahn et al. (1961) employed cytodiagnostic routinely and regarded it as suitable for the differentiation of leukoplakia, into 4 categories. King and Coleman (1965) found that the presence of keratinization did not interfere with cytodiagnostic evaluation. Waechter (1978) stated that exfoliative cytology was a valuable tool in the early diagnosis of oral leukoplakia. Tiecke and Blozis (1966), and Sandler et al. (1960) proposed that the prior removal of the keratinized layer would facilitate the cytological evaluation of hyperkeratotic leukoplakia. In contrast many authors (Silverman 1959, Silverman et al. 1958, Umiker et al. 1960, Gardner 1964, Shafer and Standish 1965, Bánóczy 1960*a*, *b*, Pape 1970, Mehta et al. 1971) believed that since the superficial keratinized layer may prevent the emergence of the deep-seated dyskeratotic cells onto the surface, cytological techniques are of little value except in leukoplakias of the fissured, ulcerated type.

We have carried out cytological studies of leukoplakias since 1958. For this reason the number of smears examined is not identical with the number of patients covered in our follow-up study.

The purpose of our cytological studies was:

1. to establish the degree and pattern of keratinization, and its relationship to the clinical type, and

2. to examine the value of cytological examination in the detection of malignant changes developing in leukoplakia, by comparison with the histological findings.

For cytological examination, scrapings were taken from the surface of the lesion with a spatula. The scraping was spread on a slide, fixed immediately in ethanol-ether and stained by our modification of Papanicolaou's method (Bánóczy 1958, 1960*a,b*, 1961*a,b*, 1968). For quantitative evaluation, 100 cells were counted in each smear. Examination for malignant change included the following features: enlargement of cell and nucleus, alteration of nuclear/cytoplasmic ratio, irregularity of nuclear membrane, nucleolar enlargement, hyperchromatism, alteration of the chromatin structure, changes in staining reaction, orangeophilia.

STUDIES OF THE KERATINIZATION PATTERN IN ORAL LEUKOPLAKIA

Examination of 250 smears from leukoplakias showed alterations in the proportion of different cell types. Regardless of the site of the lesion, cells staining yellow or red, i.e. keratinized cells, increased in number compared with the proportions found in normal oral mucosa (Trott and Bánóczy 1962) (Table 42; see Figs 9, 10 and 45 as well as colour photo 8). Statistical evaluation showed a highly significant increase in the percentage mean value of yellow cells (Table 43).

Examination of the smears for qualitative differences revealed that the shapes and sizes of the cells were very varied. Although all cells included in the scrapings were of superficial origin, their cytological appearance was markedly polymorphic. A few cells were large, round or oval (cyanophilic) or red (acidophilic—eosinophilic) in colour, but small, partly anucleated red cells, and small, shrunken, nucleated or anucleated yellow cells were considerably more numerous. The keratinized cells formed a near amorphous mass, having lost their normal shape. The nucleus was usually dark stained with one or two nucleoli.

In some of the smears the large cyanophilic and acidophilic cells contained distinct cytoplasmic granules, which were identified as keratohyaline granules. These were larger and more numerous than in normal epithelial cells. The cells with conspicuous cytoplasmic granulation usually had smaller and darker nuclei than the others.

The exfoliative cytological examination of leukoplakia gave indication of the keratinization pattern of the lesion. The presence of large, nucleated cells with keratohyaline granules amongst many shrunken, predominantly anucleated, fully keratinized cells indicated orthokeratosis or hyperorthoker-

Table 42

Distribution of keratinized cells in 250 smears from healthy oral mucosa and leukoplakia

Oral region	Cell types	Percentage of cell types	
		in leukoplakia	in normal mucosa
Hard palate	blue	5	11
	red	10	27
	yellow	85	62
Soft palate	blue	31	87
	red	41	10
	yellow	28	3
Buccal mucosa	blue	53	83
	red	22	12
	yellow	25	5
Dorsum of the tongue	blue	25	53
	red	27	32
	yellow	48	15
Gingiva	blue	20	46
	red	27	33
	yellow	53	21

Table 43

Mathematical–statistical evaluation of differences in the incidence of keratinized cells in healthy oral mucosa and leukoplakia

Oral region	Leukoplakia x_1	Normal mucosa x_2	t	p	Degree of significance
			(140)		
Hard palate	85	62	18.4	0.001	highly significant
Soft palate	28	3	13.00	0.001	highly significant
Buccal mucosa	25	5	31.00	0.001	highly significant
Dorsum of the tongue	48	15	9.2	0.001	highly significant
Gingiva	43	21	25.5	0.001	highly significant

atosis (Figs 43 and 45). In parakeratosis or hyperparakeratosis, there were mostly shrunken, yellow cells with preserved nuclei, and keratohyaline granules were negligible or absent (Fig. 44 and see colour photo 8) (Bánóczy 1968, 1971).

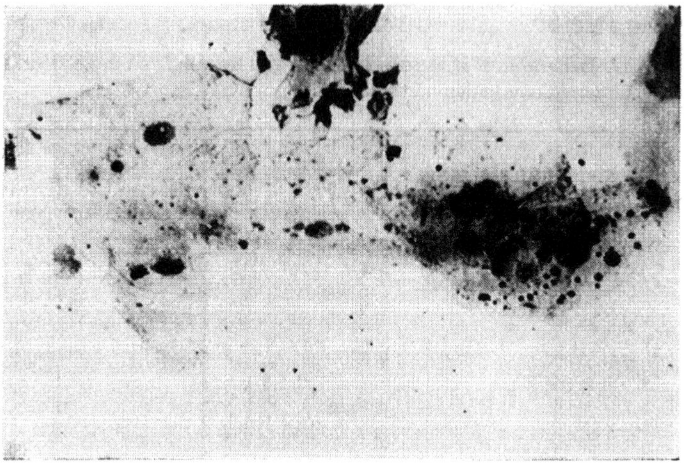

Fig. 43. Cytological appearance of buccal leukoplakia simplex. Presence of a few anucleated, keratinized cells and occurrence of a few keratohyaline (→) granules in the larger nucleated cells indicates orthokeratosis. Papanicolaou's stain, ×340

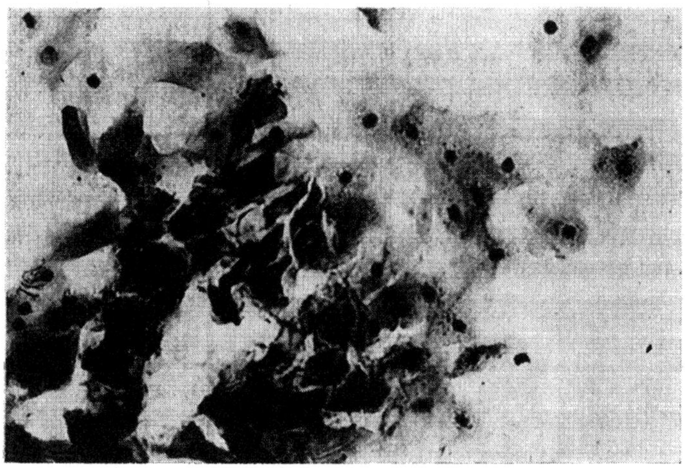

Fig. 44. Cytological appearance of verrucous leukoplakia of the tongue. Keratinized cells with shrunken nuclei; parakeratosis (→). Papanicolaou's stain, ×340

Comparison of the cytological findings with the pattern of keratinization observed histologically in each case showed that pure hyperorthokeratosis and pure hyperparakeratosis was satisfactorily detected by cytology. If,

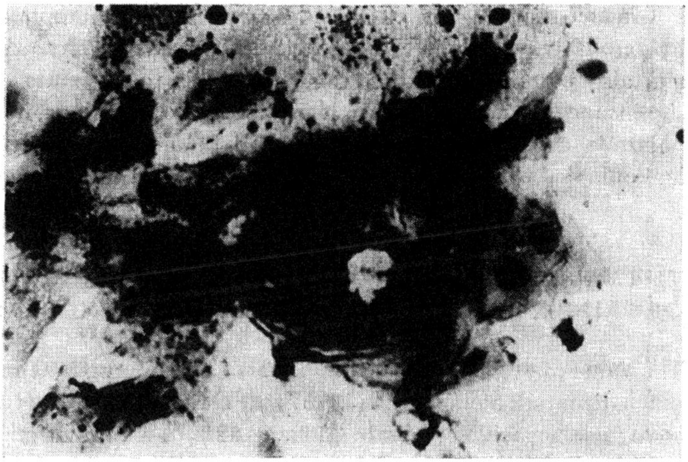

Fig. 45. Cytological appearance of verrucous plus erosive leukoplakia of the soft palate. Keratinized yellow cells admix with cells of the stratum granulosum containing many large keratohyaline (→) granules: orthokeratosis. Papanicolaou's stain, ×340

however, both keratinization patterns were present in combination in the histological sections, nearly one-third of the smears revealed only the hyperparakeratotic change (Bánóczy 1968, 1971). One possible explanation is the limited tendency to desquamation in orthokeratosis which has been substantiated at the ultrastructural level by Plackova et al. (1971).

The keratinization patterns are correlated with the clinical types of leukoplakia in Table 44 (Bánóczy 1968, 1971).

Among the simple leukoplakias, 71% were orthokeratotic, while 79% of the erosive leukoplakias were parakeratotic. A mixed ortho-parakeratotic pattern was found in a similarly low proportion of both clinical types.

Table 44

Correlation of the cytologically detected keratinization type with the clinical type

Clinical type of leukoplakia	Orthokeratosis %	Parakeratosis %	Ortho- and parakeratosis %
Simplex	71	17	12
Verrucous	48	39	13
Erosive	4	79	17

The fact that the keratinization pattern of oral leukoplakia is recognizible by exfoliative cytology gives deeper insight into the keratinization process, and also permits some indirect conclusions to be made on its prognostic significance. In accordance with the histological findings, hyperparakeratosis points to a proliferative tendency and as such is prevalent in the erosive leukoplakia, which is generally regarded as a frankly precancerous lesion.

THE VALUE OF CYTODIAGNOSTICS IN THE DETECTION OF CANCER DEVELOPMENT FROM ORAL LEUKOPLAKIA

The value of cytology in the diagnosis of malignant transformation has been much disputed. Mehta et al. (1970) and Dabelsteen et al. (1971) found that it gave false negative results in 63.9 and 62% of examinations, respectively, of hyperkeratotic leukoplakia. However, initially neither these authors nor others had taken into consideration the clinical type of leukoplakia (Bánóczy 1960*a*, *b*, 1961*a*, *b*, 1968, 1969*a*, *b*). In earlier cytological studies we found signs indicative of malignancy in 3.5% of the cases at first examination, and in 8% on re-examination. The cytological study was generally more efficient in erosive leukoplakia than in other types (Bánóczy 1961*a*, *b*, 1968, 1969*a*, *b*).

The fact that cytological evidence of malignancy was obtained in the most erosive leukoplakias with carcinomatous change, but only in a few hyperkeratotic leukoplakias undergoing malignant transformation, substantiates the observations of Silverman et al. (1958), Umiker et al. (1960) and Gardner (1964). This suggests that cytological studies are conclusive only in the fissured, erosive forms of leukoplakia. However, in our clinical experience (Bánóczy and L. Sugár 1972), the great majority of malignant transformations occur precisely in that type. This appears to define the category in which exfoliative cytology is both important and conclusive.

Cytological findings need to be reinforced by parallel histological examination to be of complete diagnostic value. Many authors have investigated oral leukoplakia by a comparative cytological and histological approach (Dabelsteen et al. 1971, Hahn 1962*b*, Mehta et al. 1970, Pomeranz and Stahl 1953, Shklar et al. 1968, Silverman and Ware 1960, Silverman et al. 1977), and have formed conflicting opinions as to the efficiency of cytology. None of them have, however, taken into consideration the difference in clinical types of leukoplakia in their evaluation (Bánóczy 1972, 1975, 1976, Bánóczy et al. 1974, Bánóczy and Rigó 1976).

To arrive at more reliable conclusions, we correlated the results of our comparative cytological and histological analysis with the clinical type of leukoplakia.

A total of 201 smears from patients with leukoplakia were stained according to Papanicolaou, and were divided into three groups according to the following criteria: (*a*) absence of abnormal or atypical cells — normal smear; (*b*) presence of a slight cellular and nuclear enlargement, slight hyperchromatism, slightly prominent nucleoli, slightly irregular nuclear membrane and increased nuclear/cytoplasmic ratio — atypical (but non-malignant) smears; (*c*) marked alteration of the nuclear/cytoplasmic ratio, pronounced, hyperchromatism, alteration of chromatin structure, altered staining affinity, orangeophilia and presence of differentiated and undifferentiated malignant cells — malignant smear (Reddy and Kameswari 1974) (see Fig. 48 and colour photo 10).

Sections obtained from the donors of the smears were evaluated as (*a*) plain leukoplakia if a non-malignant hyperkeratotic change was found, (*b*) atypical or dysplastic leukoplakia if the histological appearance satisfied the criteria outlined in chapter IV, and (*c*) malignant, if histological indications of an in situ or invasive carcinoma were demonstrable.

As to clinical type, the group studied included, respectively 58, 61 and 82 cases of simple, verrucous and erosive leukoplakias.

The cytological and histological changes were then examined for any relationship with one another and with the clinical type.

The cytological and histological findings are compared in Table 45. 151 smears were evaluated as plain leukoplakia; of these 118 (78 %) proved to be "plain" histologically. Epithelial dysplasia, carcinoma in situ and invasive carcinoma were detected in 28 (19 %), 2 (1 %) and 3 (2 %) of the remaining cases.

Twenty-six smears were classified as atypical; of these 10 (39 %), 12 (46 %) and 4 (15 %) were identified histologically as plain leukoplakia, epithelial dysplasia and invasive carcinoma, respectively. Malignant cells were detected

Table 45

Correlation of the cytological and histological findings

Cytological findings / Histology	Normal leukoplakia		Atypia		Carcinoma in situ		Invasive carcinoma		Totals	
	No.	%	No.	%	No.	%	No.	%	No.	%
Normal leukoplakia	118	78	28	19	2	1	3	2	151	100
Atypia	10	39	12	46	—	—	4	15	26	100
Malignant	3	8	2	8	2	8	18	76	24	100
Totals	130		42		4		25		201	

Table 46

Correlation of the cytological and histological findings with the clinical type

Histological findings	Normal			Atypia			Carcinoma in situ			Invasive carcinoma			Total
	Clinical type of leukoplakia												
Cytology	I.	II.	III.	I.	II.	III.	I.	II.	III.	I.	II.	III.	Total
Papanicolaou													
I–II	56	35	29	1	13	14	—	—	2	—	1	2	153
III	1	5	2	—	5	7	—	—	—	—	—	4	24
IV–V	—	1	1	—	—	2	—	1	1	—	—	18	24
Totals	57	41	32	1	18	23	—	1	3	—	1	24	201

cytologically in 24 cases; of these, invasive carcinoma and carcinoma in situ were verified histologically in 18 (76%) and 2 (8%) cases, respectively, while in two cases (8%) there were false positive findings from lesions diagnosed histologically as "plain" leukoplakia.

Correlation of the cytological and histological findings with the clinical type of leukoplakia is shown in Table 46. *Cytological and histological findings coincided in 56 (96.5%) of the 58 simple leukoplakia, in 41 (67.2%) of 61 verrucous leukoplakias and in 59 (71.9%) of 81 erosive lesions.*

To summarize, the comparative cytological and histological findings were identical in 76.6% of leukoplakias, and in 82.8% of carcinomas. False positive results were obtained in 1.3% of the cases.

Analysis of the cytological and histological findings in relation to the clinical type showed that a false negative result was frequent in verrucous leukoplakia; consistent results were obtained in only 67.2% of the verrucous lesions. Cytological examination was, however, more efficient in the erosive category, where it gave results which corresponded to the histological findings in 71.9% of the cases, and most conclusive in simple leukoplakia, where 96.5% of the cases were recognized cytologically as such. However, in that latter group the development of carcinoma was not observed.

In our experience, cytological studies have generally been more efficient than reported by other authors. The percentage of our false negative results, (23.4% among 201 patients) is much lower than the 63.8 and 62% reported by Dabelsteen et al. (1971) and Mehta et al. (1970). Our favourable results probably can be explained by the relative benignity of simple leukoplakia and the high proportion of erosive lesions (41%) in our patients. The greater efficiency of cytological examinations in erosive leukoplakias is well known (Figs 46–51 and colour photos 9–10). We agree with Mehta et al. (1970) and

Fig. 46. Carcinoma developed from erosive buccal leukoplakia which had first been observed four years earlier. The patient, a 36-year-old man, was a habitual smoker, had sharp-edged molars and bit his cheek

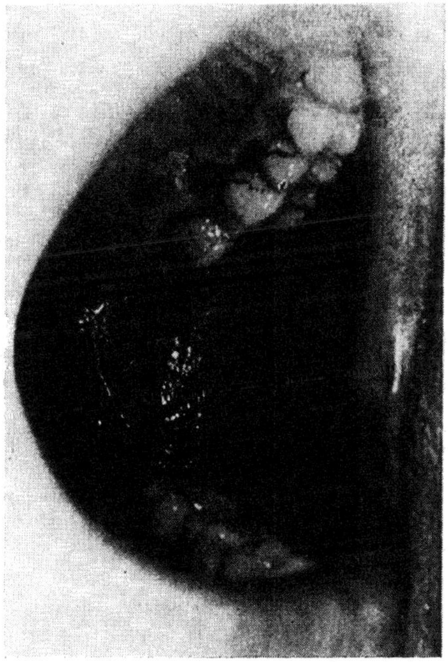

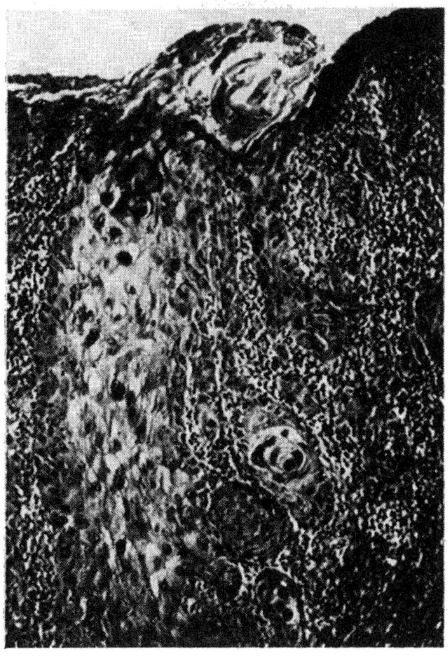

Fig. 47. Microscopic appearance of the neoplasm shown in Fig. 46: squamous cell carcinoma. H. & E., ×125

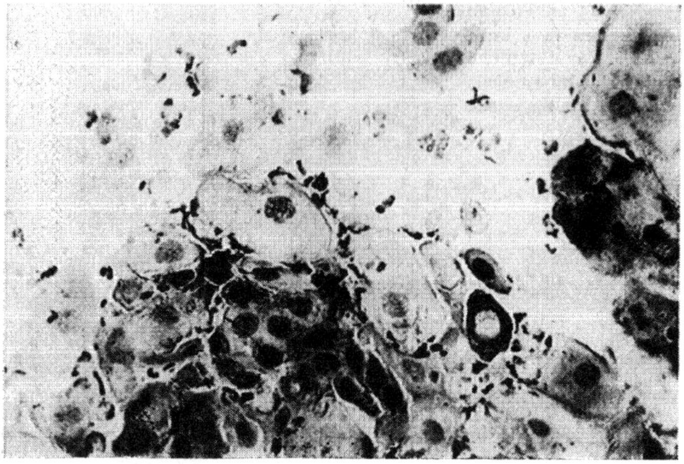

Fig. 48. Cytological appearance of the neoplasm shown in Fig. 46. Cellular polymorphism, anisocytosis, shift of the nuclear/cytoplasmic ratio. Papanicolaou's stain. ×340

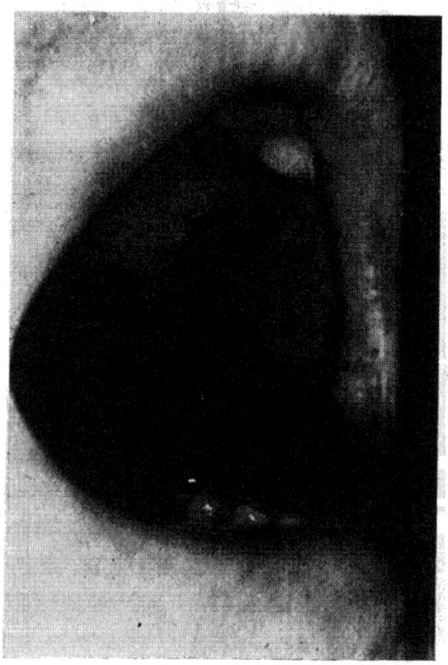

Fig. 49. Site of the carcinoma shown in Fig. 46, eight years later. Surgical excision of the lesion, radiation therapy, extraction of the molars, and stopping the smoking habit resulted in complete healing

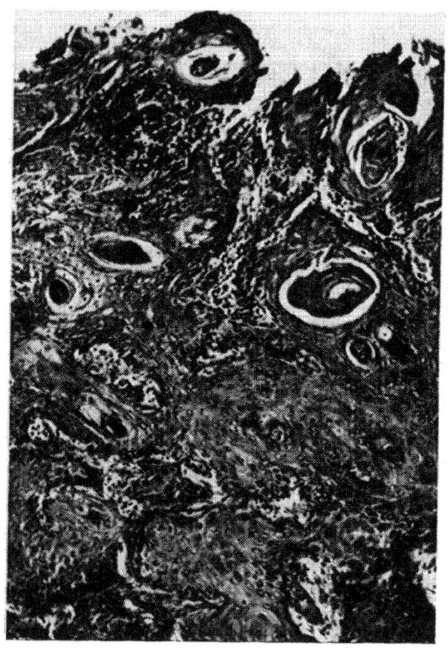

Fig. 50. Microscopic appearance of the neoplasm shown on colour photo 9: keratinizing squamous cell carcinoma. H. & E., ×125

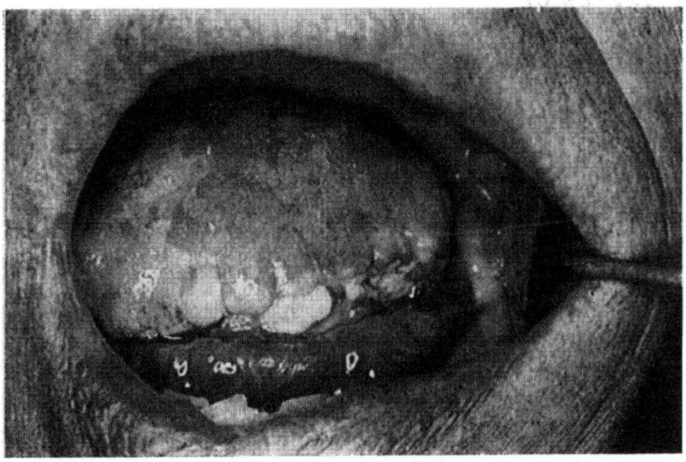

Fig. 51. The lingual lesion shown on colour photo 9, six years after surgical excision and radiation treatment. The patient died at the age of 54 years, six years after the identification of oral malignancy of metastatic carcinoma

Dabelsteen et al. (1971) that hyperkeratotic (especially verrucous) leukoplakias are difficult to identify by cytological methods, but we should like to re-emphasize their value in the diagnosis of malignant transformation in erosive leukoplakia (Bánóczy and Sugár 1972, Bánóczy 1977).

It should again be pointed out that the cytological findings are not conclusive in themselves, but only in combination with histological evidence. The fact that cytological examinations are easily repeated and the biopsy site can be selected makes them a useful tool in the diagnosis of leukoplakia.

CHAPTER VI

ELECTRON MICROSCOPIC STUDIES OF ORAL LEUKOPLAKIAS

Ultrastructural studies of the oral mucosa were begun by Sognnaes and Albright in the late fifties, first in mice (Sognnaes and Albright 1956) and later in humans (Sognnaes and Albright 1958, Albright 1960). It was shown that keratinization of the oral mucosa was not as complete as that of the skin, but was more pronounced than in any other mucosa. Since then many authors have investigated the ultrastructural characteristics of the keratinizing and non-keratinizing regions of oral mucosa (Zelickson 1961, Zelickson and Hartmann 1962, Haim 1964), and have compared it with the skin (Fasske and Themann 1959, Haim 1964, Hashimoto et al. 1966), but a detailed description of their findings is beyond the scope of this monograph. The keratinizing and non-keratinizing regions of normal human oral mucosa differ in various ultrastructural features, as listed below:

- shape and position of the basement membrane (Haim 1964, Luzardo-Baptista and Garcia-Tamayo 1968, Frithiof 1969),
- number and shape of cytoplasmic processes (Haim 1964, Frithiof 1969, 1971),
- position of desmosomes (Luzardo-Baptista and Castejon 1968, Frithiof 1971),
- shape and size of intercellular spaces (Haim 1961, Frithiof 1971),
- presence of peripheral cytoplasmic condensation (Hashimoto et al. 1966, Frithiof 1970, Luzardo-Baptista and Garcia-Tamayo 1971*a*, *b*),
- cellular glycogen content (Morgenroth and Themann 1962, Hashimoto et al. 1966, Silverman 1967, Hashimoto 1971, Silverman et al. 1971),
- presence and numbers of keratohyaline granules and tonofilaments (Hashimoto et al. 1966),
- presence and numbers of Odland bodies (membrane-coating granules) (Odland 1960, Matoltsy and Parakkal 1965, Frithiof and Wersäll 1965, 1966, Luzardo-Baptista and Castejon 1969, Luzardo-Baptista and Garcia-Tamayo 1071*c*, El-Labban and Kramer 1974*a*, *b*),
- functional differences (Luzardo-Baptista and Garcia-Tamayo 1971*c*, Squier 1970, Hayward 1973).

Electron microscopic examination of human oral leukoplakias was first reported by Themann (1958) and Fasske et al. (1958), and later by Frithiof (1963). Their cases showed no indication of malignancy at the light microscopic level, but electron microscopically both a quantitative increase in numbers and polymorphism of the mitochondria, reminiscent of cancer cells, were found, together with a lesser degree of vacuolization, but more numerous fibrillar elements in comparison to cancer cells. Barucchi et al. (1963) observed cytoplasmic vacuolization and degeneration of the mitochondria in histologically severe forms of oral leukoplakia. In a comparative ultrastructural analysis of leukoplakia and normal keratinizing oral epithelium, Haim (1964) found marked differences between the normal and pathological patterns of keratinization. In the latter the processes of the basal cells were shorter and less well-defined than in eukeratinization, the size and position of tonofilaments and keratohyaline granules were altered, and there was a shift in the normal 1:1 ratio of filamentous to amorphous elements, as occurs in dyskeratosis. Hashimoto et al. (1968) stressed the importance of the keratohyaline granules and associated tonofilaments, and of ribonucleoprotein particles in the process of keratinization. Silverman (1967) compared the ultrastructural characteristics of ten leukoplakias with those of normal oral mucosa, and related them to the light microscopic features. The ultrastructure of leukoplakia differed from that of the normal oral mucosa by the presence of stratification and discontinuity in the basement membrane, a quantitative increase of cell organelles, the appearance of striated granules in the upper part of the stratum spinosum, the formation of fibrils, the presence of keratohyaline granules, and the appearance in the stratum corneum of cells packed with an electron-dense fibrillar material, separated from one another by irregularly dilated intercellular spaces filled with a mucinous substance. J. Sugár (1968) included the examination of five labial leukoplakias in his ultrastructural studies of precancerous lesions of human skin, lip and pharynx, and concluded that destruction of the basement membrane and micro-invasion demonstrable at the ultrastructural level had commenced during the pre-neoplastic stage.

The greatest number of samples, 21 specimens of normal and 48 specimens of pathological oral mucosa (hyperplasia, leukoplakia, carcinoma), was used in the comparative ultrastructural studies of Frithiof (1969). These included investigations of the behaviour of basement membrane (Frithiof 1969), basement membrane-associated structures (Frithiof 1971), cytoplasmic membrane (Frithiof 1971), and cytoplasmic processes (Frithiof 1972) in normal tissue and in precancerous lesions or carcinoma.

Existing observations of the electron microscopic appearance of normal and pathological subcellular structures can be summarized as follows:

The basement membrane is normally continuous, of practically uniform thickness (300 to 900 Å), and separated from the basal cells by the lamina lucida. The thickness of the basement membrane tends to decrease as keratinization increases. Similar alterations are also seen in hyperplasia. Severe inflammation may cause detachment of the basement membrane from the basal cells, followed by its discontinuity, fragmentation and occasionally also by the formation of accessory basement membranes. Discontinuity and multiplication of the basement membrane can also occur in the different types of oral leukoplakia (Silverman 1967, Frithiof and Wersäll 1968). The basement membrane may be defective or even absent in invasive carcinoma. Frithiof (1969) distinguished two types of basement membrane: a thin multiple form and a thick, atypical, filamentous form. Fasske et al. (1958) suggested that the basement membrane may remain preserved in carcinoma.

Among the *structures associated with the basement membrane,* the hemidesmosomes do not differ between normal keratinizing and non-keratinizing oral epithelium. In invasive and carcinoma in situ the desmosomes are missing if the basement membrane is absent, they appear normal if the basement membrane is multiple, and they occur in varying numbers if it is atypical. Most fibrils are attached to desmosomes, thus they are, missing along with the non-periodic fibres, if the basement membrane is absent or atypical, but present if it is multiple.

The *cytoplasmic processes* of the normal epithelium are of two types (Frithiof 1971), either a broad-based structure containing tonofilaments forming desmosomes, or a narrower process without tonofilaments, which do not serve as junction with other cells. Non-keratinizing epithelium shows towards the surface (from below outward) a decrease in the number of desmosomes, and an increase in thin processes, but no processes are formed by basal cells. In keratinizing epithelium both types of processes are more numerous, and the broad-based functional processes tend to increase in number towards the surface. The junctions formed by this type of process have been described by Luzardo-Baptista and Garcia-Tamayo (1971*a*, *b*) as "macula adherens". The cytoplasmic processes of the basal cell differ from those forming intercellular junctions. The basal cells of the non-keratinizing epithelium have a flat surface devoid of processes while those of the keratinizing epithelium carry several processes of the broad type (Frithiof 1971). In invasive or pre-invasive carcinoma the normal cytoplasmic processes vary in shape and size, and abnormal processes are also present. Frithiof (1971) distinguished three types among the abnormal processes, which occur chiefly in the basal region: (*a*) proliferating cytoplasmic processes devoid of tonofilaments, but occasionally containing ribosomes; (*b*) long, thin processes containing tonofilaments, not associated with basement membrane; (*c*) processes surrounded by basement membrane residues, located adjacent to cells devoid of ribosomes. Luzardo-Baptista and Garcia-Tamayo (1971*a*, *b*) described the intercellular junctions found in pathological conditions (dysplasia and carcinoma) as zonula occludens and zonula adherens. Silverman (1967) observed a quantitative increase in desmosomes in oral leukoplakia.

In normal conditions the *intercellular space* is wider between basal cells and spinous cells than between cells of the upper flattened layers. Increase in the width of the intercellular spaces above normal signifies a pathological alteration (Haim 1964). Desmosomes of dyskeratotic cells eventually disappear (Sato and Seiji 1973). J. Sugár and Faragó (1967) observed the same in precancerous lesions of the pharynx.

A *peripheral condensation of the cytoplasm* in keratinizing epithelial cells has been described by several authors (Hashimoto et al. 1966, Frithiof 1970, Luzardo-Baptista and Garcia-Tamayo 1971*a*, *b*). Frithiof observed this phenomenon in non-keratinizing cells, but to a lesser degree. In normal non-keratinizing epithelium the peripheral cytoplasmic condensation is limited to certain regions of the superficial layer, while in the keratinizing epithelium it takes place in cells beneath the stratum corneum during the final stage of differentiation which follows upon the release of the contents of the Odland bodies into the intercellular space. Frithiof (1970) also saw a similar change in epithelial hyperplasia.

The structural features of the tonofilaments are directly related to the degree of keratinization; the greater the keratinization, the thicker the tonofilaments (Silverman 1967), which also then appear in the basal layer. The increase in the number of tonofilaments is also proportional to changes in the mitochondria (loss of the lamellar structure). In dyskeratosis, aggregations of tonofilaments appear in the suprabasal cells (Sato and Seiji 1973). The tonofilaments merge to form tonofibrils in the central and upper rows of cells in keratinizing epithelium. In abnormal conditions of keratinization (Haim 1964) the tonofilaments are localized circumferentially at the cell periphery rather than in a radial position.

It is clear that keratohyaline granules are involved in keratinization, but their role is still not fully understood. Such granules characteristically occur in the keratinizing epithelium. In abnormal conditions of keratinization they vary greatly in shape and size (Haim 1964), and in leukoplakia they first appear in the upper part of the stratum spinosum, in association with tonofilaments and ribosomes. Kempson (1974) proposed three criteria for the morphological classification of keratohyaline granules, i.e. shape, quantity of associated tonofilaments, and amount of material composing the granule.

The *bodies described by Odland* (1960) in keratinizing epithelium were independently observed by Frithiof and Wersäll (1965) and Matoltsy and Parakkal (1965); these authors named them "membrane-coating granules". Their presence was later substantiated by several other investigators (Silverman 1967, Luzardo-Baptista and Castejon 1969, Luzardo-Baptista and Garcia-Tamayo 1971*a, b*). Certain authors demonstrated acid phosphatase activity (Wolff and Holubar 1968, Luzardo-Baptista and Garcia-Tamayo 1971*c*), others (Ohashi et al. 1973) an acid mucopolysaccharide content in the Odland bodies, to which they attributed different functions in keratinizing and non-keratinizing epithelium (Squier 1970, Hayward 1973). Frithiof and Wersäll (1965) established that Odland bodies are equally present in ortho- and parakeratosis, in the form of granules 0.1 μ in diameter, located in the upper layer of the stratum spinosum. El-Labban and Kramer (1974*a*) suggested that membrane-coating granules are not independent cytoplasmic processes of keratinizing epithelium. They hold the view that the dense structures found in the intercellular spaces are also associated with cell processes, and that the cytoplasmic micro-granules which occur in non-keratinizing epithelial cells are related to cross-sections of cytoplasmic processes (El-Labban and Kramer 1974*b*).

Recent investigations have concentrated on the identification of the ultrastructural characteristics of the well-defined clinical and histological types of oral leukoplakia. Schenk (1975) reported that leukoplakias classified histologically as dysplastic exhibited, at the electron microscopic level, the changes described by Frithiof (1971) as typically precancerous. However, since previous ultrastructural studies have not covered all the internationally acceptable clinical types of oral leukoplakia (Bánóczy and L. Sugár 1972, Pindborg 1971), nor all its different histological types (dysplastic and non-dysplastic) (Bánóczy and Csiba 1970, 1972, 1976*a, b*), it seemed worth-while to analyze in parallel the light and electron microscopic appearances with regard to the clinical type (Bánóczy et al. 1978), and to employ newer ultrastructural procedures, such as stereology, morphometry (Klein-Szántó et al. 1976, Bánóczy et al. 1977, Schroeder et al. 1978), and scanning electron microscopy, to obtain more precise information.

The transmission electron microscopic, stereological-morphometric and scanning electron microscopic studies conducted in our group of patients with leukoplakia are described in the next parts of this chapter.

TRANSMISSION ELECTRON MICROSCOPIC (TEM) STUDIES

Specimens for transmission electron microscopic (TEM) examination were obtained from 12 patients with oral leukoplakia (nine men and three women), aged 35–60 years. Five cases were simple leukoplakia, two verrucous and five erosive (Bánóczy et al. 1980).

Biopsies were taken under local (nerve block) analgesia with 2% Lidocaine, using a 4 or 5 mm corneal (punch), or a scalpel. In each case, part of the biopsy was processed for light microscopic examination. The excised tissue intended for transmission electron microscopy was fixed in 2.5% glutaraldehyde, washed in pH 7.3 Na-cacodylate, postfixed in 2% OsO_4 (pH 7.2) as described by Palade (1952), dehydrated in step-graded ethanol, and embedded in Durcupan. Ultra-thin sections were counter-stained with 5% uranyl acetate and lead citrate, and examined in a TESLA RS 500 electron microscope.

The following investigations were pursued:

1. The identification of possible ultrastructural characteristics that could be related to the clinical type and histological appearance of oral leukoplakia.

2. The detection of possible ultrastructural indications of cancer in lesions recognized by light microscopy as dysplastic.

Simple leukoplakia

Most lesions classified clinically as simple leukoplakia showed on light microscopic examination epithelial hyperplasia, acanthosis, ortho- or hyperorthokeratosis, a well-developed granular layer, a very mild inflammatory cell

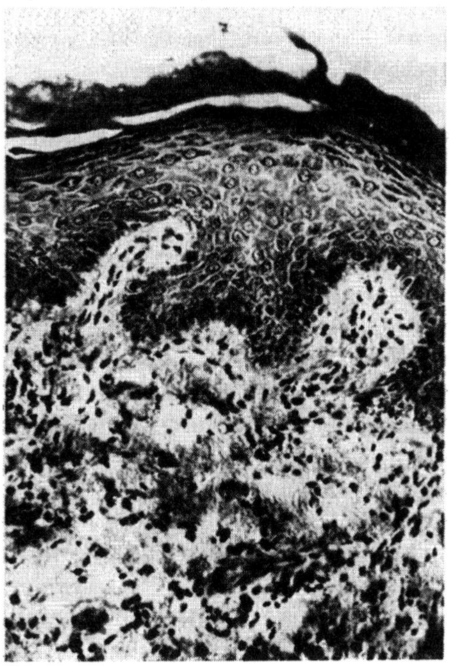

Fig. 52. Light microscopic appearance of simple leukoplakia. Epithelial hyperplasia, acanthosis, hyperorthokeratosis, conspicuous stratum granulosum, and slight inflammatory cell reaction in the connective tissue. H. & E., ×125

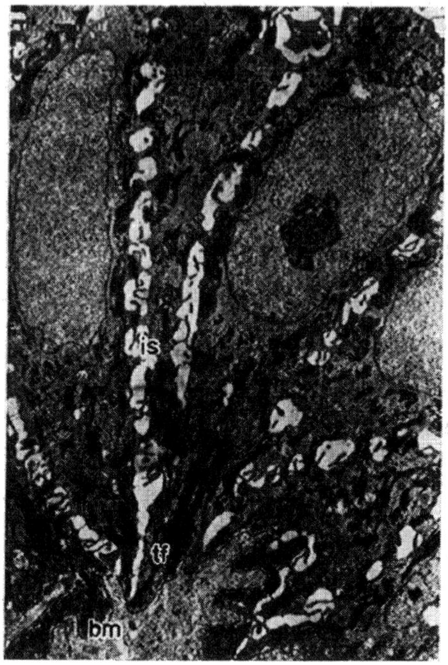

Fig. 53. Basal layer of epithelium in simple leukoplakia: The tonofilaments merge to form a homogeneous dense substance, ordered into bundles. The intercellular spaces are dilated, the basement membrane is intact. bm = basement membrane, tf = tonofilament, is = intercellular space. ×5,700

reaction in the connective tissue, and sharp demarcation of the latter from the epithelium (Fig. 52).

By electron microscopy the *basement membrane* was as a rule continuous, and well-preserved, but with considerable variations in its thickness; in places it showed multiplication (Figs 53–55) and failed to follow the contours of the cytoplasmic processes (Fig. 55). Most hemidesmosomes were intact (Figs 53 and 55).

Stratum basale. Most basal cells extended many processes, predominantly of the broad type (Figs 53 and 54) containing tonofilaments in conjunction with hemidesmosomes (Fig. 53). Two pathological forms of processes were observed, one a ribosome-containing structure, devoid of tonofilaments (Figs 53 and 54), the other a tonofilament-containing one not associated with basement membrane (Fig. 55). No hemidesmosomes occurred in these atypical locations. The nuclei of the basal cells were round or oval, and the nuclear membrane showed a slightly undulating contour in places. The cytoplasm contained bundles of condensed tonofilaments, ribosomes, and mitochondria which showed loss of structural definition (crystolysis; Fig. 54) in places.

Stratum spinosum. The cellular and nuclear volume both tended to increase toward the surface and the nuclei were round or slightly oval, with an undu-

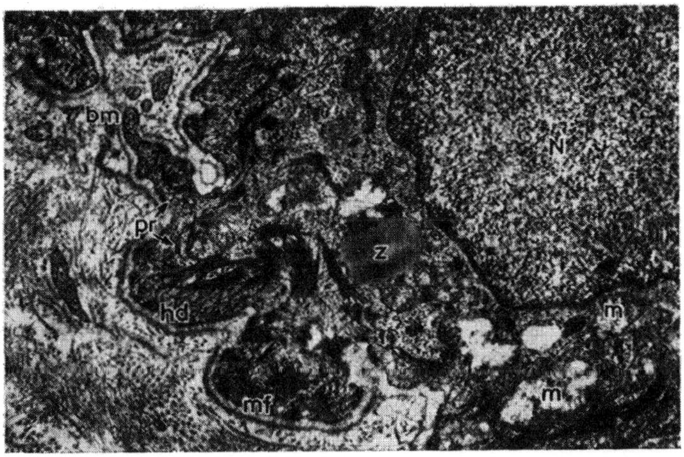

Fig. 54. Basal cell from oral epithelium in simple leukoplakia. The basement membrane is preserved at the interface between epithelium and connective tissue, but in places it shows thickening, ramifications, and multiplication. The microfibril connections of the basement membrane with the cytoplasmic membrane of the basal cell are easily visible throughout, but especially in the region of the hemidesmosomes. The cell contains a few deteriorating mitochondria, and a lipid granule. Most processes of the basal cell arise on a broad base, but some atypical processes, without tonofilaments, containing, however, ribosomes can also be seen. bm = basement membrane, hd = hemidesmosomes, mf = microfibril, m = mitochondrion, l = lipid granule, pr = cytoplasmic processes. ×15,000

lating nuclear membrane (Figs 56 and 58). The nuclear chromatin was evenly distributed (Figs 56 and 58), the nucleoli were enlarged and increased in number to 3 or 4 per cell (Fig. 58).

The cytoplasmic tonofilaments formed bundles located not infrequently at the cell periphery like a "crown of thorns" (Fig. 57). The number of tonofibrils increased toward the upper layers of the stratum spinosum (Figs 57 and 58), and the peripheral tonofibrils formed junctions with desmosomes (Fig. 59). The cytoplasm contained many ribosomes which decreased in number toward the superficial layers. Most mitochondria appeared intact, but in the superficial layers they were less numerous and increasingly showed indications of degeneration (crystolysis, rhexis; Figs 57 and 58).

Stratum granulosum. The cells contained thick, condensed tonofibrils (Fig. 60) and in places electron-dense keratohyaline granules (Figs 60 and 61) with aggregations or ribosomal clumps at their periphery (Fig. 60). No mitochondria were found, but lipid granules were occasionally present (Fig. 61). The nuclei were flat and elongated with condensed chromatin substance (Fig. 61).

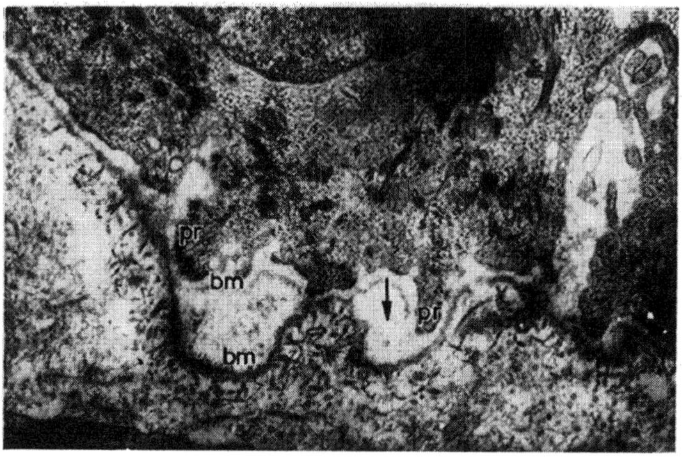

Fig. 55. Simple leukoplakia. The basement membrane shows ramification, duplication and thickening at the epithelial–connective tissue interface, and does not always follow the contours of the cytoplasmic processes (→). Note splitting of the microfilaments at the sites where the basement membrane has receded. bm = basement membrane, pr = cytoplasmic processes. ×21,000

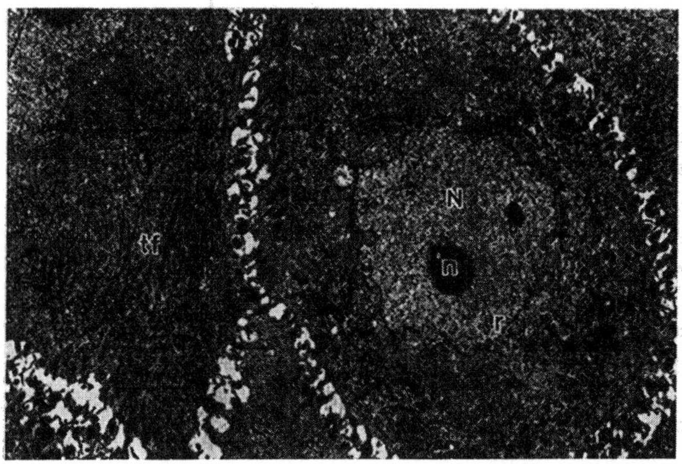

Fig. 56. Stratum spinosum of oral epithelium in simple leukoplakia. The cellular and nuclear volumes both tend to increase towards the surface. The cytoplasm contains many tonofilaments and ribosomes. The nuclear membrane shows undulating contours. The nuclear chromatin is evenly distributed. N = nucleus, tf=tonofilament, n = nucleolus. ×4,500

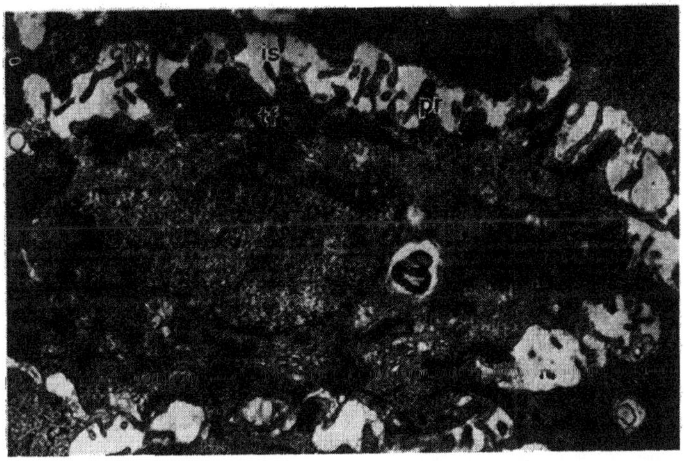

Fig. 57. Stratum spinosum of oral epithelium in simple leukoplakia. The intercellular space is dilated and the arrangement of the intracellular tonofilaments is reminiscent of a crown of thorns. is = intercellular space, tf = tonofilament, pr = cytoplasmic processes. ×9,000

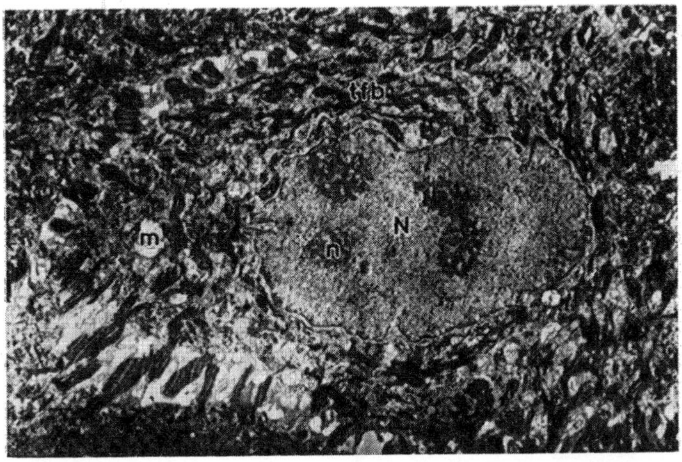

Fig. 58. Central part of stratum spinosum in simple leukoplakia. The cytoplasm contains many tonofibrils. The mitochondria are damaged (crystolysis, rhexis). Supernumerary nucleoli are present. N = nucleus, n = nucleolus, tfb = tonofibril, m = mitochondrion. ×6,000

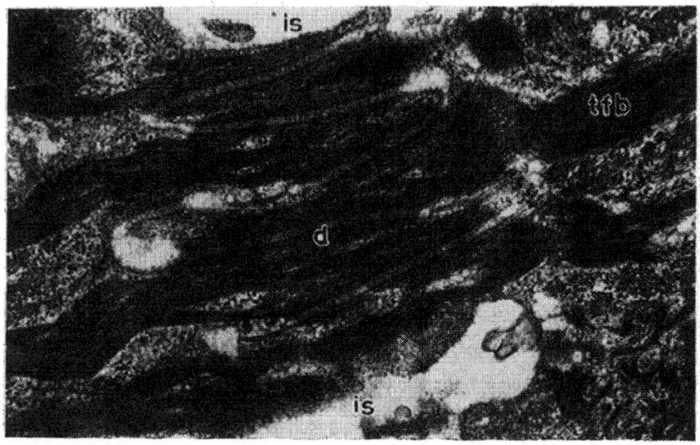

Fig. 59. Stratum spinosum in simple leukoplakia. The intercellular space is dilated, the intercellular junctions are furnished by many desmosomes. The tonofibrils form bundles which are intimately associated with the desmosomes at the cell periphery. is = intercellular space, tfb = tonofibril, d = desmosomes. ×27,000

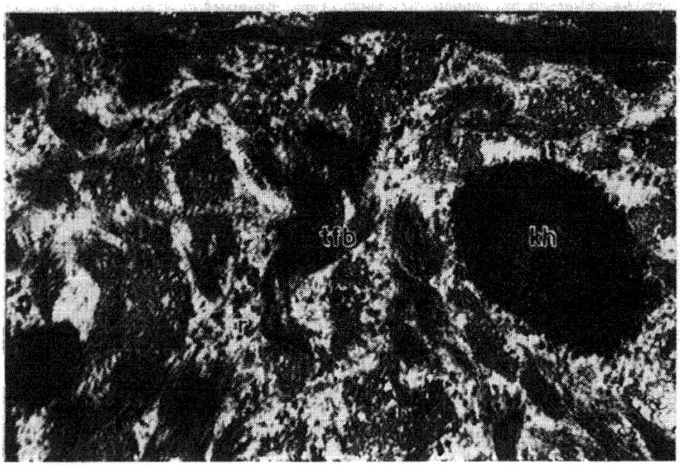

Fig. 60. Stratum granulosum in simple leukoplakia. Note aggregation of tonofibrils and ribosomes at the surface of the keratohyaline granules, kh = keratohyaline granule, r = ribosome, tfb = tonofibril. ×48,000

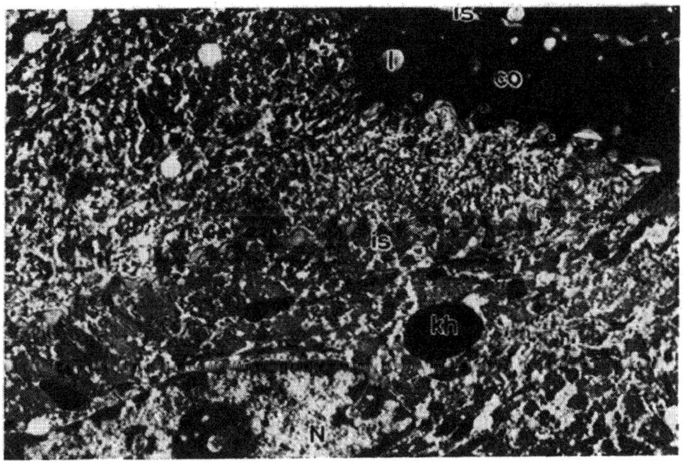

Fig. 61. Simple leukoplakia: interface between the stratum granulosum and corneum. Keratohyaline granules of varied sizes are dispersed in cells of the lower rows. The keratinized layer and the cells underneath it contain bodies reminiscent of lipid granules. co = stratum corneum, is = intercellular space, N = nucleus, kh = keratohyaline granule, l = lipid granule. ×9,000

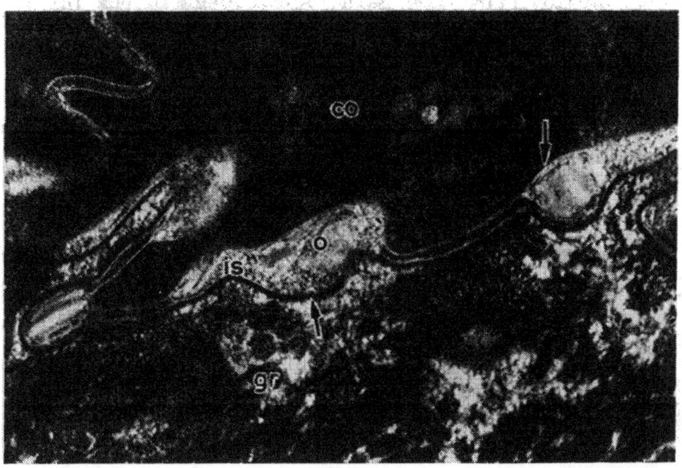

Fig. 62. Simple leukoplakia: interface between the stratum granulosum and corneum. Note peripheral condensation of the cytoplasm (→) and passage of Odland bodies into the intercellular space, gr = stratum granulosum, co = stratum corneum, is = intercellular space, o = Odland bodies. ×48,000

The intercellular spaces were narrow, and contained in places lamellar structures (Odland bodies; Fig. 62), and peripheral condensation of the cytoplasm of adjoining cells (Fig. 62).

Verrucous leukoplakia

The two verrucous lesions showed on light microscopic examination epithelial hyperplasia, acanthosis, both hyperparakeratosis and hyperorthokeratosis above a stratum granulosum, and a very slight inflammatory cell infiltration of the connective tissue. In one case there were indications of very slight dysplasia. The interface between epithelium and connective tissue was preserved in both lesions (Fig. 63).

By electron microscopy, the *basement membrane* showed both thickening and thinning, and generally did not follow the contours of the cytoplasmic membranes. Its continuity was preserved, but it was multi-layered in places, with ramifications extended between the connective tissue fibres (Figs 64 and 65). At the interface between epithelium and connective tissue, the basement membrane was attached by microfibrils to the cytoplasmic membrane of basal cells above, and to collagen fibres below (Figs 64 and 65).

Stratum basale. Most cytoplasmic processes of the basal cells were of the broad type which contain tonofilaments. A few were of the non-tonofilamentous, narrow type. The pathological forms of cell processes seen in simple

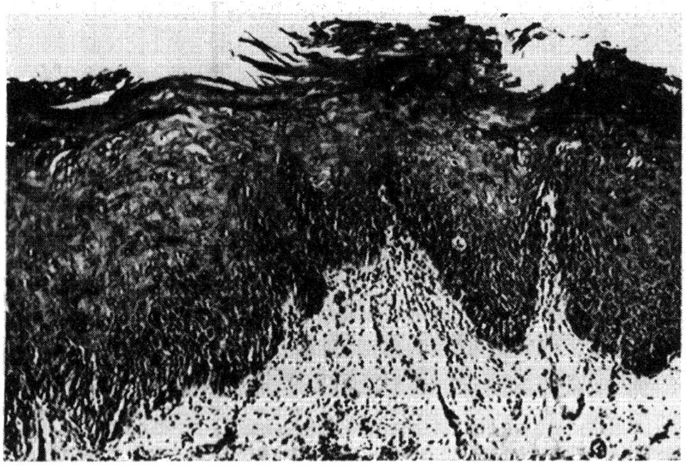

Fig. 63. Light microscopic appearance of verrucous leukoplakia. Epithelial hyperplasia, acanthosis, in some places hyperparakeratosis, in others hyperorthokeratosis above a stratum granulosum, slight inflammatory cell infiltration of the connective tissue, and a slight dysplasia. H. & E., ×125

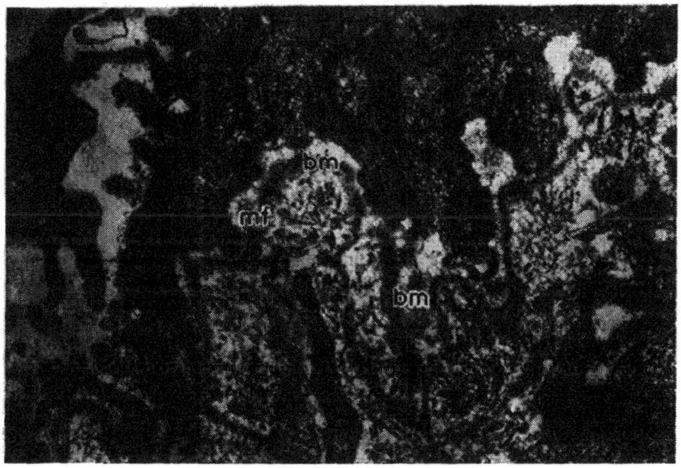

Fig. 64. Verrucous leukoplakia: epithelial–connective tissue interface. The basement membrane is thickened in some places and thinned in others, and does not always follow the contours of the cytoplasmic membrane. Its continuity is preserved, but in places it shows stratification, and branches which extend between the connective tissue fibres. bm = basement membrane, mf = microfibrils. ×21,000

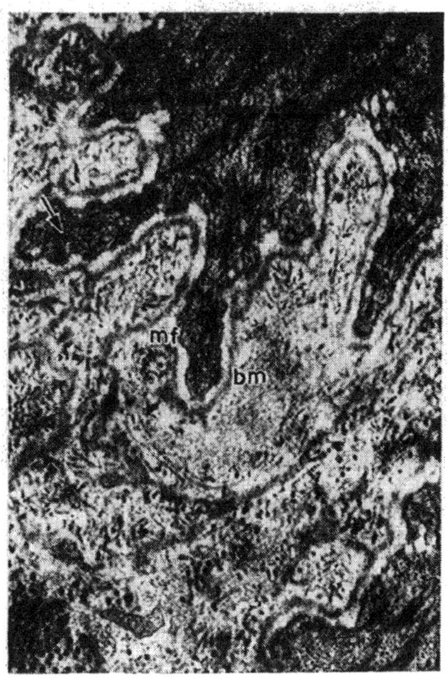

Fig. 65. Verrucous leukoplakia: epithelial–connective tissue interface. The basal cells extend narrow processes, containing tonofilaments (→), the basement membrane is multi-layered, with attaching micro-fibrils. bm = basement membrane, mf = microfibrils. ×21,000

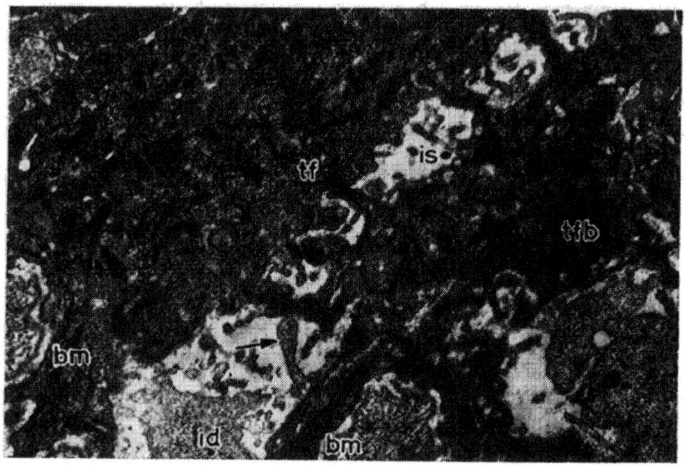

Fig. 66. Verrucous leukoplakia: basal cell. The tonofilaments have merged to form fibrils. The interdigitating intercellular junctions have drawn apart. Pseudopodial cytoplasmic processes, in places devoid of a cytoplasmic membrane (→) extend into the dilated intercellular spaces. bm = basement membrane, tf = tonofilament, tfb = tonofibril, id = intercellular debris, is = intercellular space. × 12,000

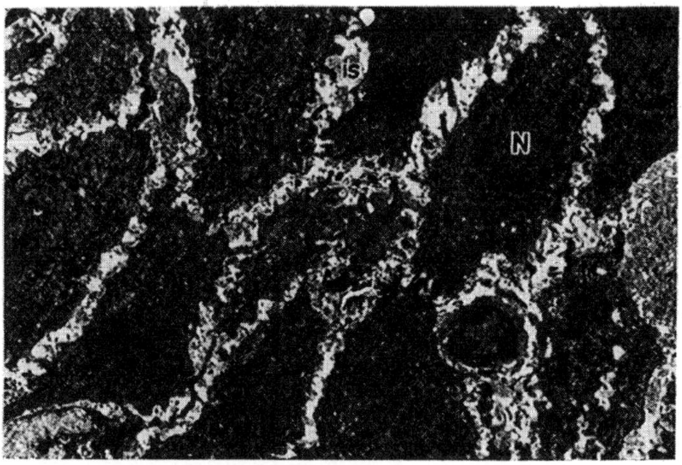

Fig. 67. Verrucous leukoplakia: stratum basale and stratum spinosum. The nuclei are lobulated, the cytoplasmic tonofilaments fused to form tonofibrils, the intercellular space is dilated. is = intercellular space, N = nucleus. ×4,200

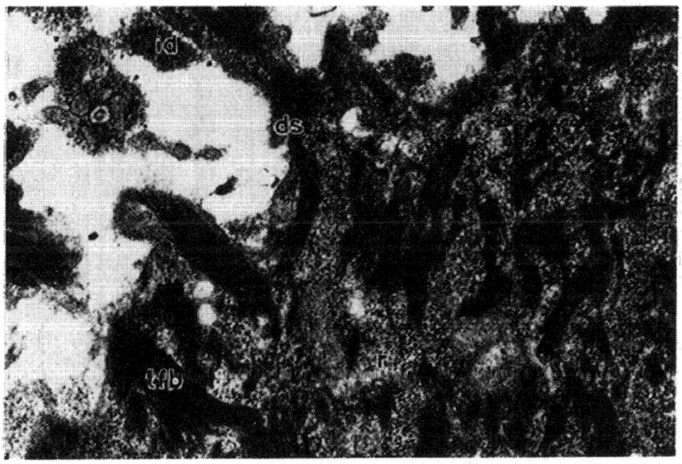

Fig. 68. Verrucous leukoplakia: central part of the stratum spinosum. The aggregated cytoplasmic tonofibrils are associated with desmosomes at the cell periphery. The ribosomes are ordered into rosettes. Some of the intercellular junctions are open, but the desmosomes appear intact. The dilated intercellular space is filled by cell debris, consisting chiefly of ribosomes. Id = intercellular debris, tfb = tonofibrils, d = desmosome, r = ribosome. ×21,000

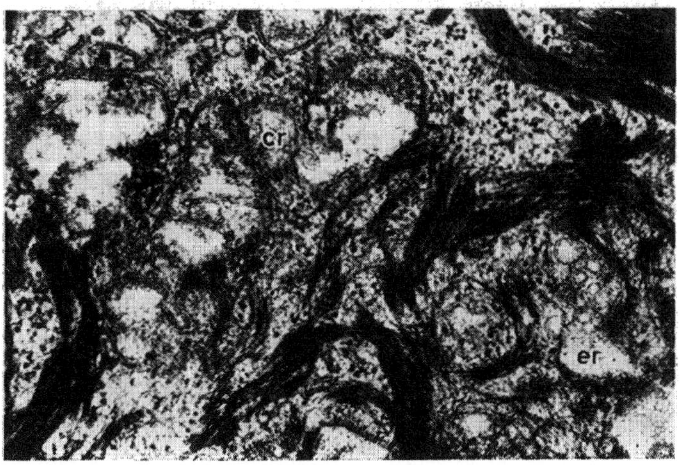

Fig. 69. Verrucous leukoplakia: superficial part of the stratum spinosum. The mitochondria show signs of cristorhexis, the endoplasmic reticulum is dilated, cr = cristorhexis, er = endoplasmic reticulum. × 36,000

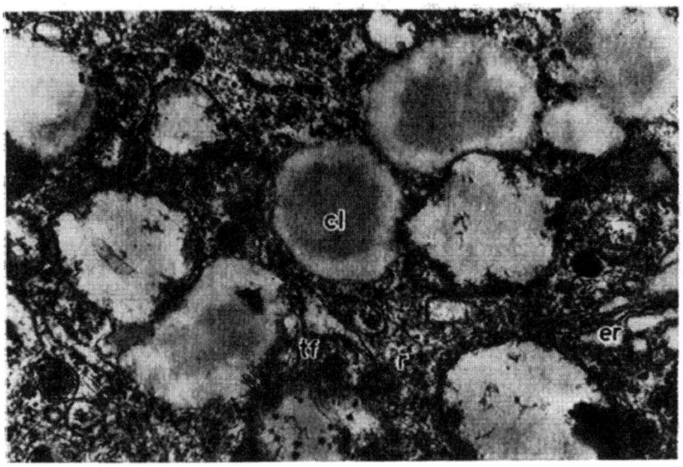

Fig. 70. Verrucous leukoplakia: superficial part of the stratum spinosum. The mitochondria show signs of cristolysis. The cisternae of the endoplasmic reticulum are dilated, the filaments fragmented, and there are few free ribosomes. cl = cristolysis, r = ribosome, er = endoplasmic reticulum, tf = tonofilaments. ×27,000

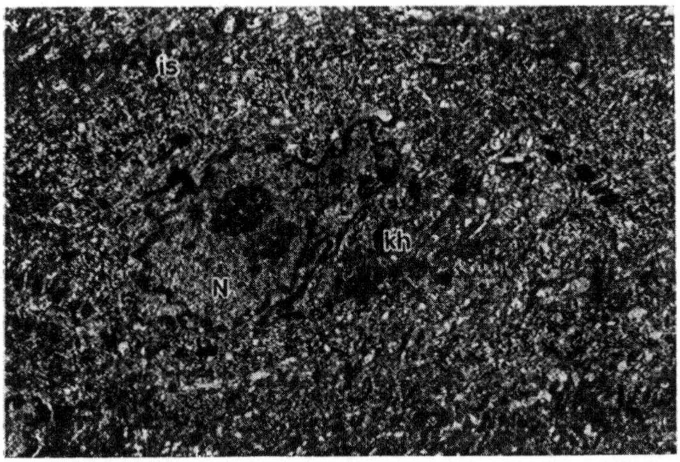

Fig. 71. Verrucous leukoplakia: stratum granulosum. Cells with and without keratohyaline granules alternate in this layer. The intercellular spaces are narrow. kh = keratohyaline granule, is = intercellular space, N = nucleus. ×21,000

leukoplakia were also encountered in the verrucous lesions (Fig. 66). The cytoplasmic tonofilaments fused to form tonofibrils in increasing numbers, when compared with similar cell layers of simple leukoplakia, and the interdigitated intercellular junctions were drawn apart (Figs 64 and 66). The mitochondria were generally intact, only a few appeared damaged.

Stratum spinosum. The spinous cells had lobular nuclei (Fig. 67). The cytoplasmic tonofilaments were either condensed and homogeneous, or broken, and some of them were aggregated at the cell periphery (Fig. 68). The intercellular spaces were widened. Ribosomes were aggregated into rosettes (Fig. 68). Most mitochondria were damaged, showing signs of cristolysis and rhexis (Fig. 69). The endoplasmic reticulum was dilated in all cell layers (Fig. 70).

Stratum granulosum. Cells either containing or devoid of keratohyaline granules were alternately present in one row. Those without granules had a wreath-like peripheral condensation of tonofilaments which in places formed a homogeneous mass (Figs 71 and 72); these were attached to desmosomes. Of the cytoplasmic organelles the ribosomes and mitochondria showed a decrease in number, and the latter also exhibited signs of cristolysis. The

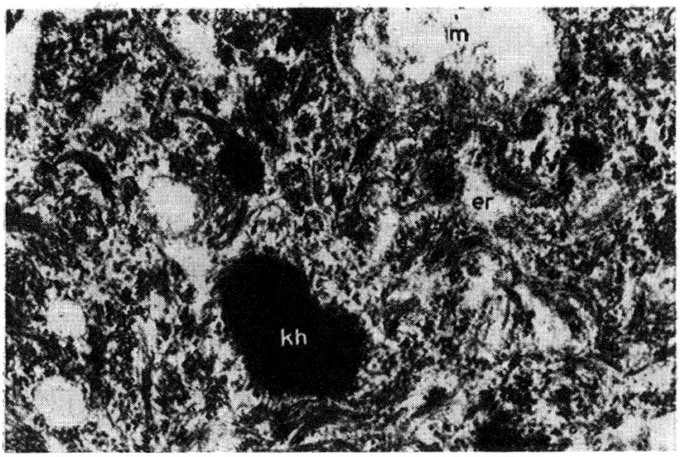

Fig. 72. Verrucous leukoplakia: stratum granulosum. The keratohyaline granules are intimately associated with ribosomes and tonofibrils. The endoplasmic reticulum is markedly dilated. er = endoplasmic reticulum, kh = keratohyaline granules, m = mitochondrion devoid of cristae. ×36,000

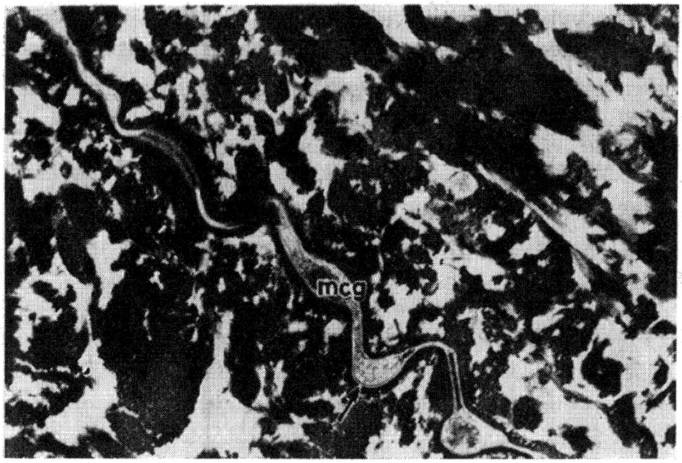

Fig. 73. Verrucous leukoplakia: stratum granulosum. Note peripheral condensation of the cytoplasm (→), and release of membrane-coating granules into the intercellular space. mcg = membrane-coating granule. ×27,000

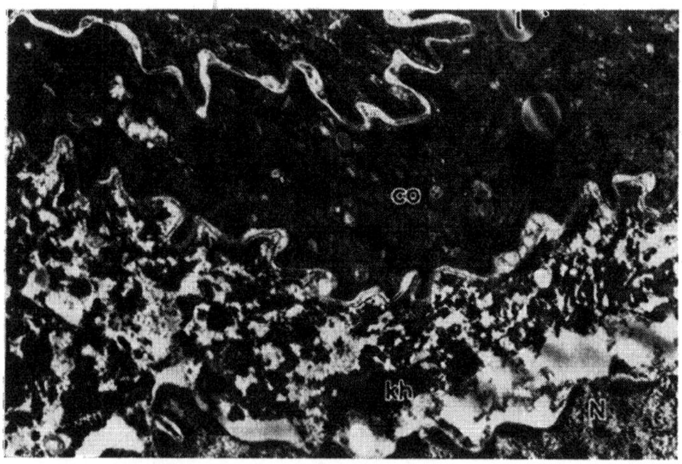

Fig. 74. Verrucous leukoplakia: interface between the stratum granulosum and corneum. The cell contains homogeneous, dense tonofibrils, but all other organelles have deteriorated. co = stratum corneum, N = nucleus, l = lipid granule, kh = keratohyaline granule. ×27,000

nuclei were lobulated (Fig. 71). Intercellular spaces were narrowed. Peripheral condensation of the cytoplasm, and release of membrane-coating granules into the intercellular space were obvious (Fig. 73).

Stratum corneum. Some cells had a flattened nucleus; the cytoplasm was filled with a homogeneous, horny substance, enclosing in places lipid granules (Fig. 74).

Erosive leukoplakia

The light microscopic appearance of erosive leukoplakia was characterized by epithelial hyperplasia, superficial ulceration, parakeratosis, and moderate to severe epithelial dysplasia occurred in three of the five cases studied. The demarcation between epithelial and connective tissues was indistinct in places (Fig. 75).

By electron microscopy the *basement membrane* had a fibrous appearance, with branches extending into the superficial layer of the connective tissue, and with stratification in places. The intercellular spaces separating the basal cells were dilated and the interdigitated, intercellular junctions drawn apart. The basement membrane filled the gaps between basal cells, but it was

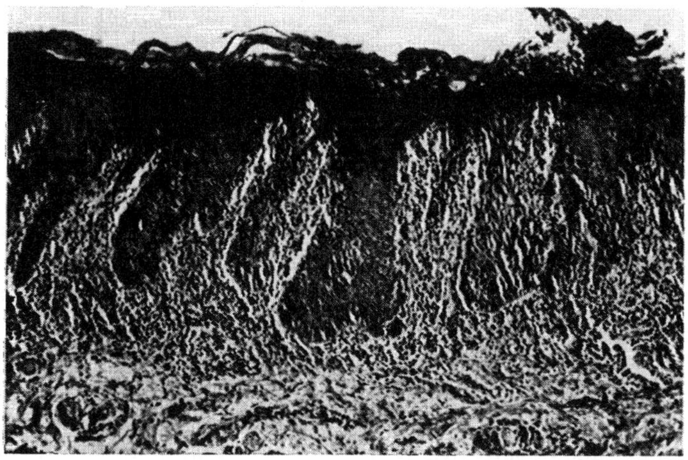

Fig. 75. Microscopic appearance of erosive leukoplakia. Note hyperplastic epithelium, parakeratosis, massive inflammatory cell infiltration of the connective tissue, and signs of severe dysplasia. H. & E., ×125

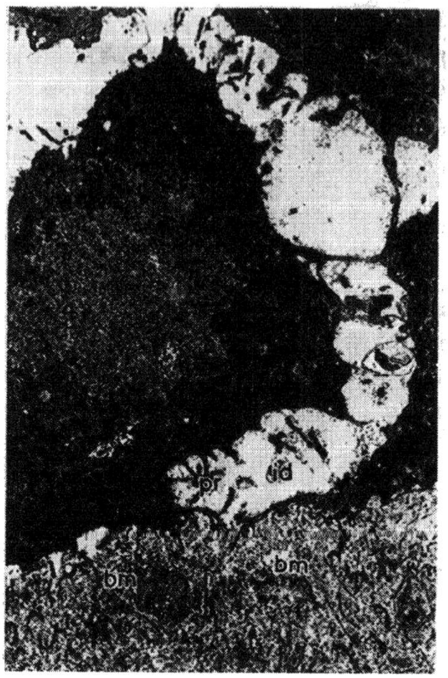

Fig. 76. Erosive leukoplakia: basal layer. The basement membrane exhibits thickening, multiplication, ramification into the superficial layers of the connective tissue, and in places discontinuity (→). At the epithelial–connective tissue interface, cytoplasmic processes are extended into the dilated intercellular space which contains cell debris consisting chiefly of ribosomes. The interdigitating intercellular junctions are all drawn apart, and most desmosomes appear damaged. bm = basement membrane, id = intercellular debris, pr = cytoplasmic processes. ×6,900

discontinuous in places; these were sites of predilection for basement membrane rupture (Fig. 76).

Stratum basale. At their laminar surface the basal cells extended the abnormal cytoplasmic processes observed in simple leukoplakia. Intact hemidesmosomes decreased in number. The basal cells contained bundles of tonofilaments, many ribosomes, and a few damaged mitochondria (Fig. 76).

Stratum spinosum. The most conspicuous change was dilatation of the intercellular space, which was associated with splitting of most intercellular junctions. The cytoplasmic membrane and processes were coated by a floccular precipitate which originated from the intercellular substance (Fig. 77).

Nuclei were lobulated with nucleoli of irregular shapes and numbers, and unevenly distributed chromatin (Figs 77 and 78). The double limiting membrane of the nucleus showed sinusoidal dilatation of the space between the two lamellae, and thickening of the inner lamella (Fig. 78).

Cells in the lower rows of the stratum spinosum contained many tonofilaments, which fused to form tonofibrils in places (Fig. 77), but these were generally less numerous than in the simple and verrucous types of leukoplakia. Ribosomes were unevenly distributed and formed aggregations (Fig. 78.) The upper rows of the stratum spinosum contained dark and clear cells (Fig. 79), which respectively, had an increased or decreased number of ribosomes.

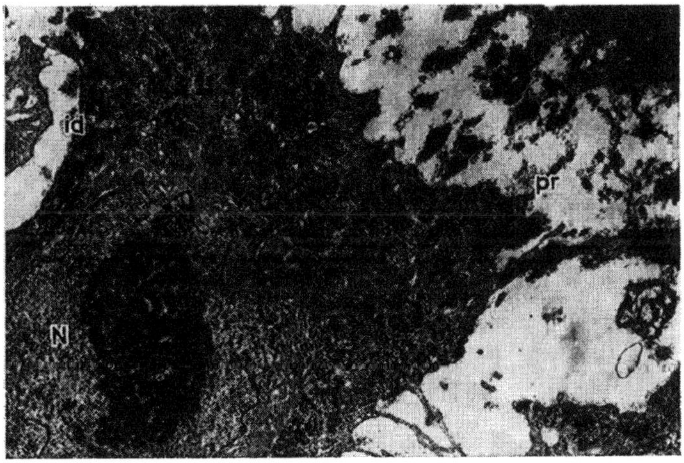

Fig. 77. Erosive leukoplakia: stratum spinosum. Most intercellular junctions are open, the intercellular spaces are dilated, and the surfaces of the cytoplasm and its processes are coated by a floccular precipitate originating from the intercellular cement substance. The intercellular space contains cross-sections of cytoplasmic processes, and cell debris, consisting chiefly of ribosomes. N = nucleus, pr = cytoplasmic process, id = intercellular debris. ×6,000

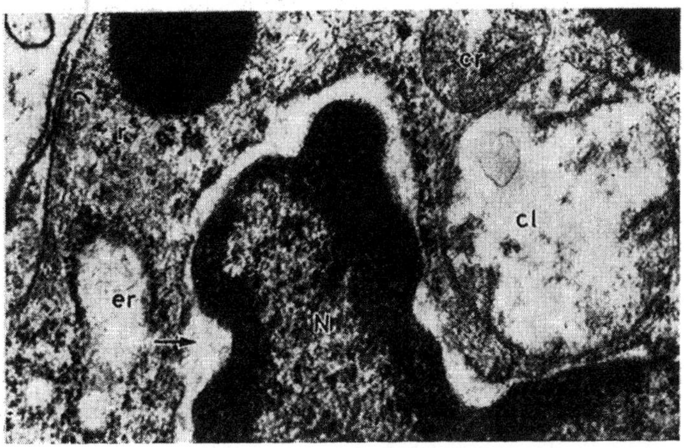

Fig. 78. Erosive leukoplakia: stratum spinosum. The nuclei are lobulated, and the space between the two lamellae of the nuclear membrane shows sinusoidal dilation (→). The inner nuclear membrane is thickened, and the bulk of the chromatin is condensed along the inner membrane. The mitochondria show signs of cristolysis and rhexis, the ribosomes are few and form rosettes, the cisternae of the endoplasmic reticulum are dilated. N = nucleus, r = ribosome, cr = cristorhexis, cl = cristolysis. ×27,000

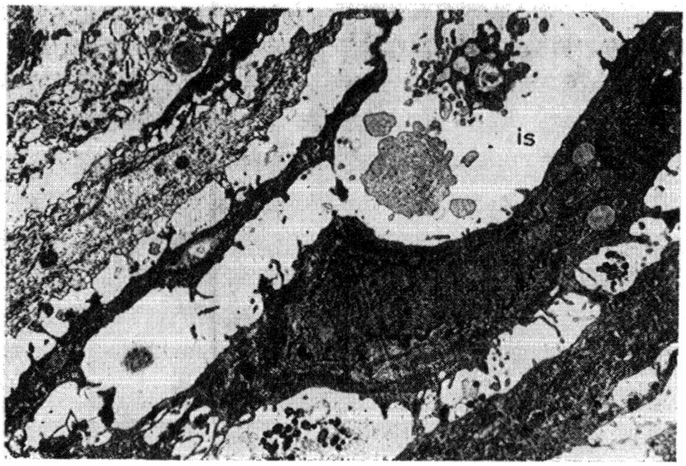

Fig. 79. Erosive leukoplakia: superficial part of the stratum spinosum. The light cells are in the process of deterioration, the dark cells contain many ribosomes. The junctions with interdigitation have disappeared; single intact desmosomes connect adjacent cells with one another. is = intercellular space, L = deteriorating light cell. ×5,700

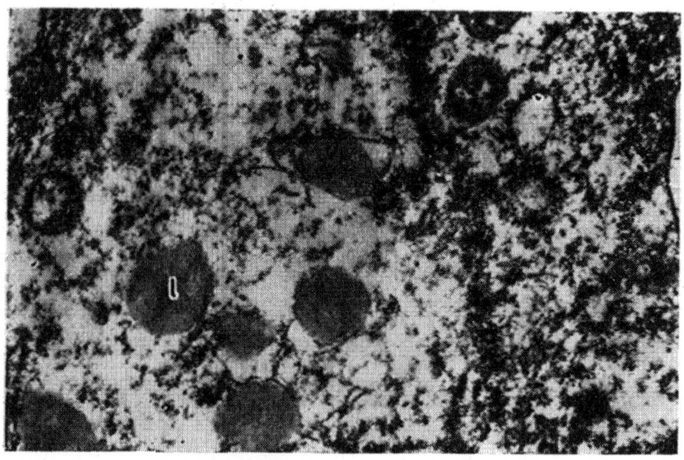

Fig. 80. Erosive leukoplakia: superficial part of the strat um spinosum. The light cell contains only few ribosomes and the mitochondria have been replaced by dense bodies which resemble lipid granul es l = lipid granule. × 21,000

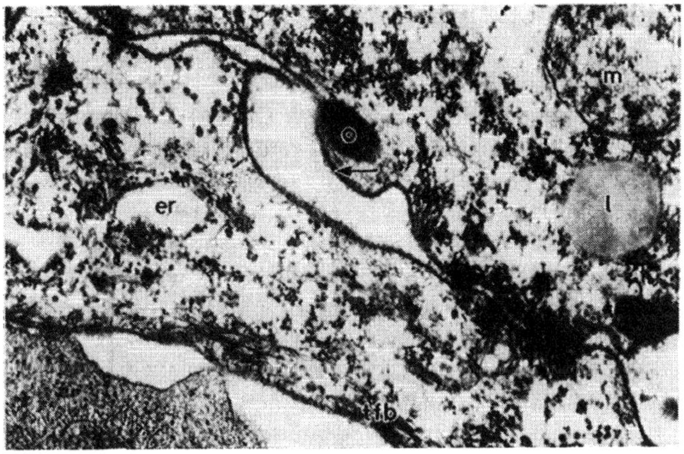

Fig. 81. Erosive leukoplakia. Note dilated endoplasmic reticulum, damaged mitochondria and presence of a lipid granule inside the pale cell. Note paucity of cytoplasmic tonofibrils, peripheral condensation of the cytoplasm (→), and Odland bodies. er = endoplasmic reticulum, m = mitochondrion, tfb = tonofibril. ×35,500

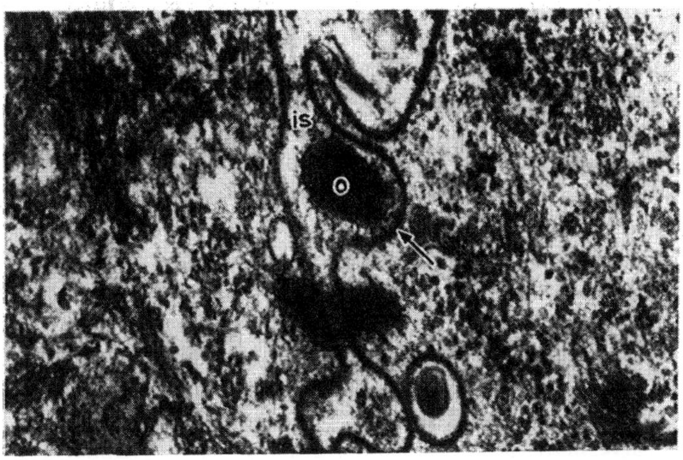

Fig. 82. Erosive leukoplakia: superficial part of the stratum spinosum. The cytoplasm is condensed along the cell periphery (→), and Odland bodies are released into the intercellular space. o = Odland body, is = intercellular space. ×66,000

Most mitochondria were damaged and were replaced by lipid granules (Fig. 80). Keratohyaline granules were sparsely present in a few cells.

Cells of the upper rows of the stratum spinosum and of the lower rows of the *stratum superficiale* contained Odland bodies and a peripheral condensation of the cytoplasm (Figs 81 and 82). In sections from non-ulcerated lesions, the upper cell rows exhibited the parakeratotic changes seen in verrucous leukoplakia.

These ultrastructural changes correspond with those described by other authors. In addition a close correlation between certain ultrastructural phenomena in the given clinical types and their different histological appearances was detected in the present studies.

The *basement membrane* was of variable thickness and occasionally multiple in all three clinical types, but while its continuity was preserved in simple and verrucous leukoplakia, it was occasionally discontinuous and obliterated in the erosive type. Hemidesmosomes were also less numerous in erosive leukoplakia. These observations in combination with the findings of Silverman (1967), J. Sugár (1968) and Frithiof (1971), suggest that erosive leukoplakia with histological evidence of epithelial dysplasia is a preneoplastic lesion.

Predominance of the broad, tonofilament-containing *cytoplasmic processes* (Frithiof 1971, Luzardo-Baptista and Garcia-Tamayo 1971*a*, *b*) was usually associated with the clinical (simple and verrucous) types that exhibited increased keratinization. Pathological processes occurred in all three clinical types of leukoplakia.

In all three types, the *intercellular spaces* were wider between basal and spinous cells than between the flat cells of the upper rows (Frithiof 1971). Dilatation of the intercellular space was, however, considerably greater in erosive leukoplakia than in the other two types. This accords well with the observation of Haim (1964), J. Sugár and Faragó (1967) and J. Sugár (1968) that the intercellular junctions are drawn apart in precancerous and cancerous epithelium.

The disposition of *tonofilaments* changed with the degree of keratinization. In simple and verrucous leukoplakia the basal cells contained many tonofilaments, which then fused to form tonofibrils in the central and upper layers (Silverman 1967) in both perinuclear and peripheral locations. This phenomenon, together with the aggregation and homogenization of tonofilaments, was most pronounced in verrucous leukoplakia, and is characteristic of dyskeratosis (Sato and Seiji 1973, Haim 1964). The reduced number of tonofilaments and keratohyaline granules found in erosive leukoplakia corresponded to the parakeratotic pattern of keratinization found in this particular clinical type. In simple and verrucous leukoplakia many keratohyaline granules, with ribosomal aggregations attaching to their surfaces, appeared in the upper part of the stratum spinosum and in the stratum granulosum but, unlike Silverman (1967), we failed to demonstrate any association between keratohyaline and tonofilaments.

Odland bodies and peripheral condensation of the cytoplasm occurred in all three clinical types of leukoplakia.

In all types, most *mitochondria* were intact in the basal cells, but tended to degeneration toward the surface.

Ribosomes were diffusely arranged in the simple type of lesion, but in the upper cell rows as well as in the more severe types they tended to increase in number and form rosettes (Schenk 1975) which, according to J. Sugár (1968), are phenomena typically associated with carcinogenesis. The dark and light (electron-dense and electron-lucent) cells seen in erosive leukoplakia had formerly been observed by J. Sugár (1968) during the development of cutaneous carcinoma. The appearance of such cells can be ascribed to damage of cytoplasmic organelles.

Nuclear changes were observed in erosive leukoplakia. The space between the double nuclear membrane showed sinusoidal dilatation, the nuclear chromatin was unevenly distributed, and the shapes and numbers of nucleoli were irregular.

It follows that in simple and verrucous leukoplakia, where the predominant histological changes are related to keratinization, the ultrastructural alterations also indicate this tendency. Thus there is enhanced tonofibril formation, an increase in the number of keratohyaline granules and Odland bodies, and obvious signs of dyskeratosis. In contrast, *the electron microscopic appearance of the histologically dysplastic, precancerous leukoplakias reveals several changes regarded as preneoplastic,* such as discontinuity of basement membrane, a decrease in the number of hemidesmosomes, pathological basal-cell processes, nuclear and nucleolar changes, degeneration of tonofilaments and mitochondria, and rosetting of ribosomes.

MORPHOMETRIC (STEREOLOGICAL) INVESTIGATIONS

Morphometric or stereological methods have among others been employed for the quantitative analysis of cell organelles. This approach can disclose important information about the interrelationships of structure and function, and such observations can be easily correlated with the results obtained by other methods, wether biochemical and/or physiological.

The basic concepts of morphometry—or more precisely, stereology—were originally developed by geologists. The quantitative study of three-dimensional systems from a two-dimensional image was originated by the French geologist Delesse in 1847. Details of the stereologic study of electron micrographs of cells were elaborated recently by Weibel (1969, 1970), Weibel and

Bolender (1973), and Weibel et al. (1966). The working concept of the method is the existence of quantitative relationships between the mean dimensions of cell organelles and their profiles seen in sections. Thus the mathematical–statistical analysis of the mean dimensions of organelles randomly measured in sections permits conclusions to draw about the real, three-dimensional structure.

During recent years quantitative data for normal oral epithelium and submucosal connective tissue have been obtained from morphometric and stereologic study of light and electron microscopic preparations from various oral sites (Schroeder and Münzel-Pedrazzoli 1970, 1973, Meyer and Schroeder 1975, Landay and Schroeder 1976, Klein-Szántó and Schroeder 1977, Bernimoulin and Schroeder 1977). This prompted us to employ morphometry for the stereologic analysis and comparative evaluation of the different types of oral leukoplakia (Klein-Szántó et al. 1976, Bánóczy et al. 1977, Schroeder et al. (1978).

The purpose of our study was to estimate stereologically the ultrastructural components of epithelial tissue from simple leukoplakia arising in two different oral sites, and to identify the morphological characteristics involved in its differentiation in comparison with normal oral epithelium.

Biopsies were taken from 17 patients with simple leukoplakia, aged 29–77 years, with a 4 mm corneal trephine, under local analgesia with 2% Lidocaine solution. In eight cases the biopsy was obtained from a buccal lesion, in nine cases from one located on the floor of the mouth (Figs 83 and 84). All biopsy donors were patients of the Clinic of Maxillo-Facial Surgery and Conservative Dentistry, Semmelweis University Medical School, Budapest, and all biopsy specimens were submitted for processing and evaluation to the Department of Oral Structural Biology, Institute of Dentistry, University of Zürich.

The specimens were fixed in 2.5% glutaraldehyde and 2% paraformaldehyde, as described by Karnovsky (1961), and each was divided into 4 to 5 blocks, about 1 mm thick, cut perpendicularly to the epithelial surface. After preliminary fixation for 2 h, the blocks were washed, fixed for another 2 h in 1.33% OsO_4, dehydrated in step-graded ethanol and embedded in Epon (Luft 1961). Sections 1–2 mm thick were cut and stained with PAS or toluidine blue–azure (Schroeder 1973).

Of the available material five and six samples derived from buccal mucosa and the floor of the mouth, respectively, proved to be suitable for further processing for histometric and stereological analysis. From each sample three blocks were selected at random for further study. Two blocks originating from the unaffected sublingual mucosa of a patient with leukoplakia, as well as existing morphometric data from normal buccal mucosa (Landay and Schroeder 1976) were used for comparative evaluations.

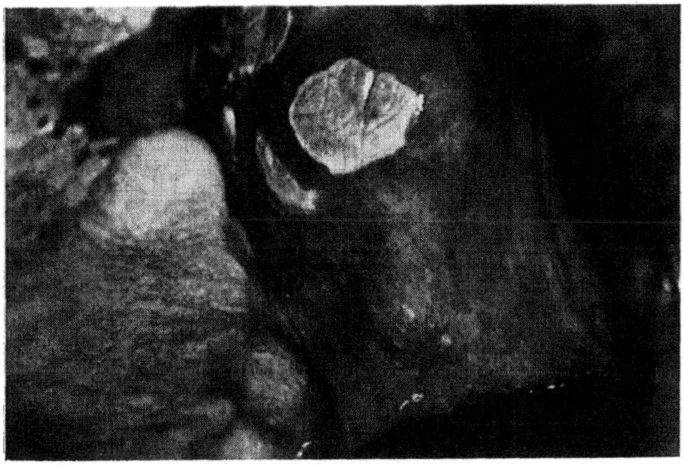

Fig. 83. Simple leukoplakia: a sharply delineated, isolated white patch on the buccal mucosa of a 55-year-old male patient

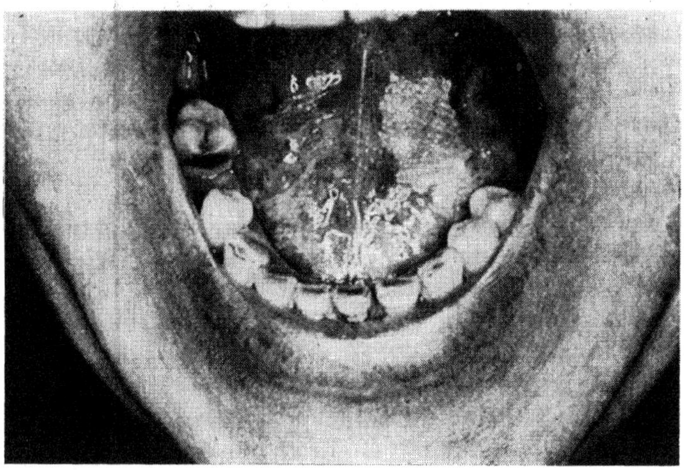

Fig. 84. Simple leukoplakia: a sharply delineated, homogeneous white patch on the floor of the mouth of a 52-year-old female patient

The thickness of the epithelium was measured in three locations on one randomly selected section from each block (Meyer and Schroeder 1975) (Table 47), using the projection screen of a Wild microscope, the mean of three measurements was taken in terms of μm.

Table 47

Comparison of the thickness of epithelium (μm) in different sites of oral leukoplakia

Site	Buccal mucosa		Mucosa of the floor of the mouth	
	leukoplakic $\bar{X} \pm S$	normal $\bar{X} \pm S$*	leukoplakic $\bar{X} \pm S$	normal $\bar{X} \pm S$**
Epithelial processes	204 ± 64	580 ± 90	157 ± 121	186 ± 45
Above connective tissue papillae	98 ± 32	240 ± 60	91 ± 80	101 ± 32
Mean	132 ± 34	480 ± 90	102 ± 42	140 ± 13
Stratum corneum	51 ± 63	—	26 ± 15	—
No. of biopsies	3	10	6	1

* Landay and Schroeder, 1976

** The standard deviation applied to different measurements within a series of section originating from the same biopsy specimen.

Ultra-thin sections were cut with an LKB ultratome. Care was taken that each section included the entire thickness of the epithelium. Sections were mounted on carbon-coated VECO copper grids, counter-stained with uranyl-magnesium acetate and lead citrate (Fraska and Parks 1965, Reynolds 1963), and examined in a Phillips EM 201 electron microscope. Electron micrographs were taken on 35 mm film suitable for morphometric analysis (Weibel et al. 1966).

For stereological analysis we used micrographs of randomly selected ultra-thin sections taken at two levels of magnification and involving five epithelial layers (Schroeder and Münzel-Pedrazzoli 1970), i.e. stratum basale, stratum suprabasale, central and upper stratum spinosum, and stratum granulosum).

At the first level, 6 electron micrographs of the stratum basale were examined at x 3,070 magnification, and then 3 micrographs each of the other strata at x 1,400. Thus 3×18 micrographs of each block, a total 594 micrographs of the two groups of leukoplakia, and 36 micrographs of normal sublingual epithelium were included in the study.

At the second level, 12 additional micrographs were prepared at $\times 6{,}070$ primary magnification from each area sampled at the first level. Thus 60 micrographs were sampled per block (total 1,980) at both levels for the leukoplakias and a total of 120 for normal sublingual epithelium.

The electron micrographs were subjected to quantitative analysis by the stereological method of Weibel and Bolender (1973). A coherent double-lattice test system was used for the morphometric estimation of cell components

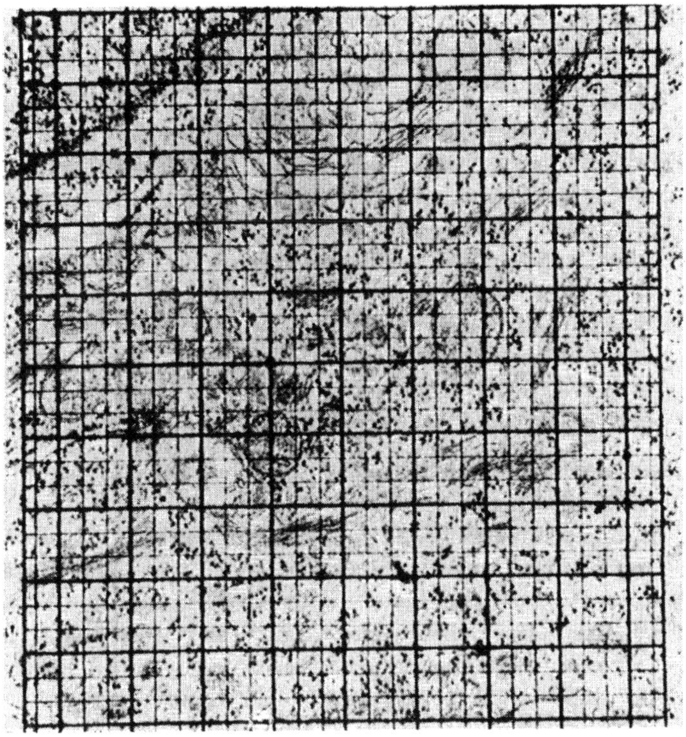

Fig. 85. Double lattice system employed for the morphometric determination of cell components, superimposed upon an electron micrograph of a leukoplakia from the floor of the mouth (at the second level of magnification) ×23,000

at both levels of magnification. The system (Weibel 1969) consisted of a triangular frame of predetermined size, which enclosed a network of heavy and light lines crossing to form 99 heavy points and 891 light ones (Fig. 85). The intersection points of the heavy lines were used for the estimation of the relative volume (V_v) of frequent and evenly distributed cell components, while those of the light lines for the quantitative determination of less frequent cell components. The intersection points of membrane profiles and heavy lines were used for the estimation of surface density (S_v). All intersection points were stored in an electronic data collector (Weibel 1969). Relative volume (V_v) and surface density (S_v) were calculated by basic stereological formulas (Weibel 1969, Weibel and Bolender 1973), where

V_v = volume density, the volume of the cell component related to unit volume (relative or fractional volume), and

S_V = surface density, the surface dimension of the cell component related to unit volume.

Raw data were averaged and transformed into stereological terms by a Hewlett-Packard 9830 calculator, which printed out the final data automatically in a tabulated form (Hammer and Schroeder 1977). For comparative purposes, all data so obtained were related to 1 cm^3 epithelial thickness or 1 cm^3 epithelial cytoplasmic volume.

The methods and results of our stereological studies have been reported in great detail in several previous publications (Klein-Szántó et al. 1976, Bánóczy et al. 1977, Schroeder et al. 1978).

General morphometric features of leukoplakic and normal epithelium

The numerical values of epithelial thickness in normal and leukoplakic oral mucosa are compared in Table 47.

In buccal leukoplakia, the epithelium was 132 ± 34 μm thick, and usually contained few connective tissue papillae. Thus the interface between epithelium and connective tissue was straight in all cases except one which had finger-like epithelial processes. Above the connective tissue papillae and in the rete processes the epithelium was on average 98 ± 32 μm and 204 ± 64 μm thick, respectively (see Table 47). The stratum granulosum was prominent, and the stratum corneum was thick (51–23 μm), owing to a homogeneous orthokeratosis.

In leukoplakia of the floor of the mouth, the epithelium showed similar characteristics to buccal leukoplakia, but its average thickness was less, 102 ± 42 μm. In this group of leukoplakias too the connective tissue papillae were few in all cases except one. Mean epithelial thickness was 91 ± 80 and 157 ± 121 μm above the papillae and within the processes, respectively (see Table 47). The stratum corneum was thinner (26 ± 15 μm) compared to buccal leukoplakia. Infiltration of the connective tissue by inflammatory cells was not a regular phenomenon in either site of leukoplakia, although minor lymphocytic infiltrations were detected in the marginal zones of a few sections. The normal buccal epithelium, examined for comparison, differed histologically from the leukoplakic epithelium, being thicker both above the papillae and within the rete processes.

The epithelium of normal sublingual mucosa was a little thicker than in leukoplakia from the same site. Histologically it consisted of a typical nonkeratinizing epithelium without a stratum granulosum and stratum corneum, and with relatively shallow connective tissue papillae.

The transition from normal to leukoplakic epithelium was abrupt and conspicuous in all strata.

Composition of the epithelial tissue

The morphometric appraisal of the composition of the epithelial tissues is shown in Figs 86–88.

Measurements of unit volume in each epithelial stratum in buccal leukoplakia indicated variations in certain components. The nuclear volume tended to decrease markedly from the lower towards the upper strata. Investigating changes of the cytoplasmic components (Fig. 86) the mitochondria and membrane-bound organelles showed a decrease in relative volume from the basal to the granular layer, while the amount of filament bundles tended to increase from the basal to mid-spinous layer The density of free ribosomes was constant in all strata except the granulosum. The density of structureless cytoplasmic ground substance (cgs) remained roughly constant in all layers except the basal one. In the latter the proportion of melanocytes and small lymphocytes (non-keratinocytes) was about 10%. The intercellular space was narrow, and of a low density in all strata; the desmosomes numbered 7 to 24 per unit area.

The structure of the leukoplakic epithelium of the floor of the mouth strongly resembled that of the buccal leukoplakia, i. e., the volume of the nucleus decreased toward the surface and also the components of the cytoplasm underwent similar changes as in buccal leukoplakia; the volumetric density of mitochondria and membrane-bound organelles gradually decreased between stratum basale and stratum granulosum while that of the bundled filaments increased up to the mid-spinous layer. Quantity of free ribosomes and density of the cytoplasmic ground substance (being 40–50% in each layer)—except for the basal layer—remained fairly unchanged. There were about 5% melanocyte and some lymphocytes in the stratum basale, the intercellular space showed low density and the number of desmosomes reached 4–21 per unit area.

Unlike leukoplakic epithelia, the normal epithelium of the floor of the mouth showed an abrupt stepwise change in the volumetric density of its components, especially from the suprabasal to the mid-spinous layer (Fig. 88). The density of the cytoplasmic ground substance showed a relative decrease, while an enormous mass of filaments filled the major part of the cytoplasm of cells located in the mid-spinous layer and superficial layers. While the cytoplasmic filaments of the basal cells formed orderly bundles, those of the suprabasal cells were divided between equal fractions of bundled filaments and single ones intertwined to form a loose network. These single filaments filled 60–70% of the cytoplasm in the higher strata, in which the size of the bundled fraction was reduced to a minimum. In the basal layer the non-keratinocytes, especially the lymphocytes, were more numerous than in other layers. In the suprabasal and upper

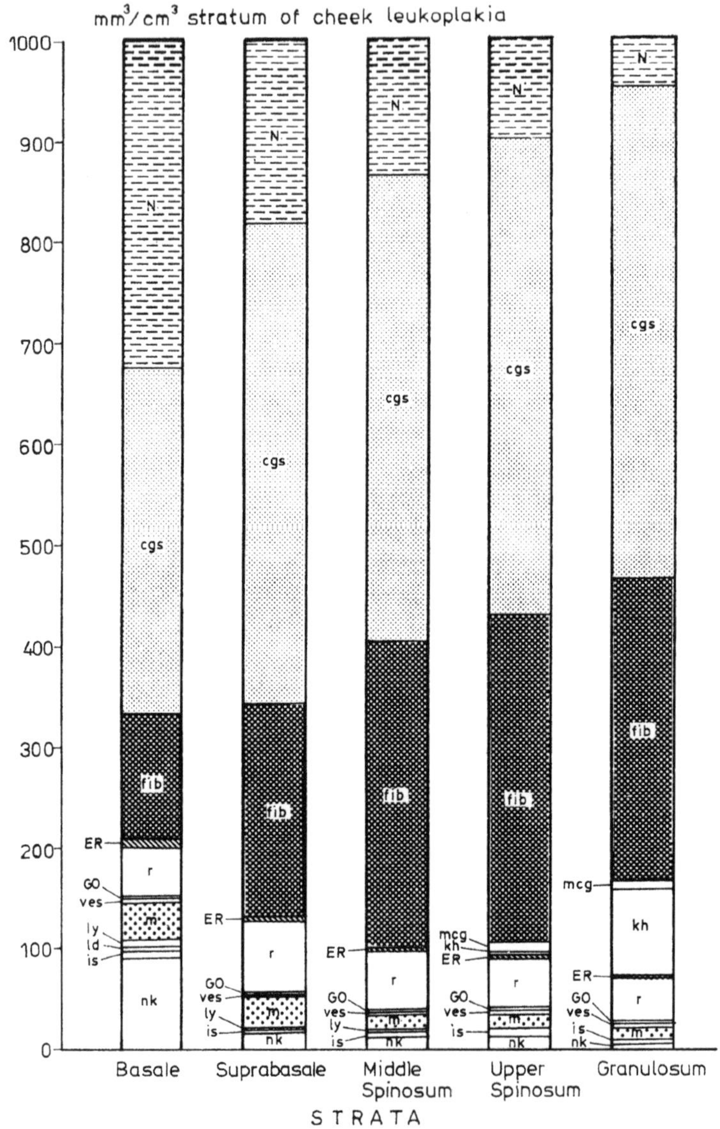

Fig. 86. Diagrammatic presentation of epithelial tissue components in buccal leukoplakia, in terms of mm³ related to 1 cm³ of each o five epithelial layers. N = nucleus, cgs = cytoplasmic ground substance, fib = filaments ordered into bundles, ER = rough surfaced endoplasmic reticulum, r = ribosomes, GO = Golgi apparatus, ves = cytoplasmic vesicles not associated with the Golgi complex, m = mitochondria, ly = lysosome-like bodies, is = intercellular space, nk = non-keratinocytes, kh = keratohyaline granules, mcg = membrane-coating granule, ld = lipid droplets

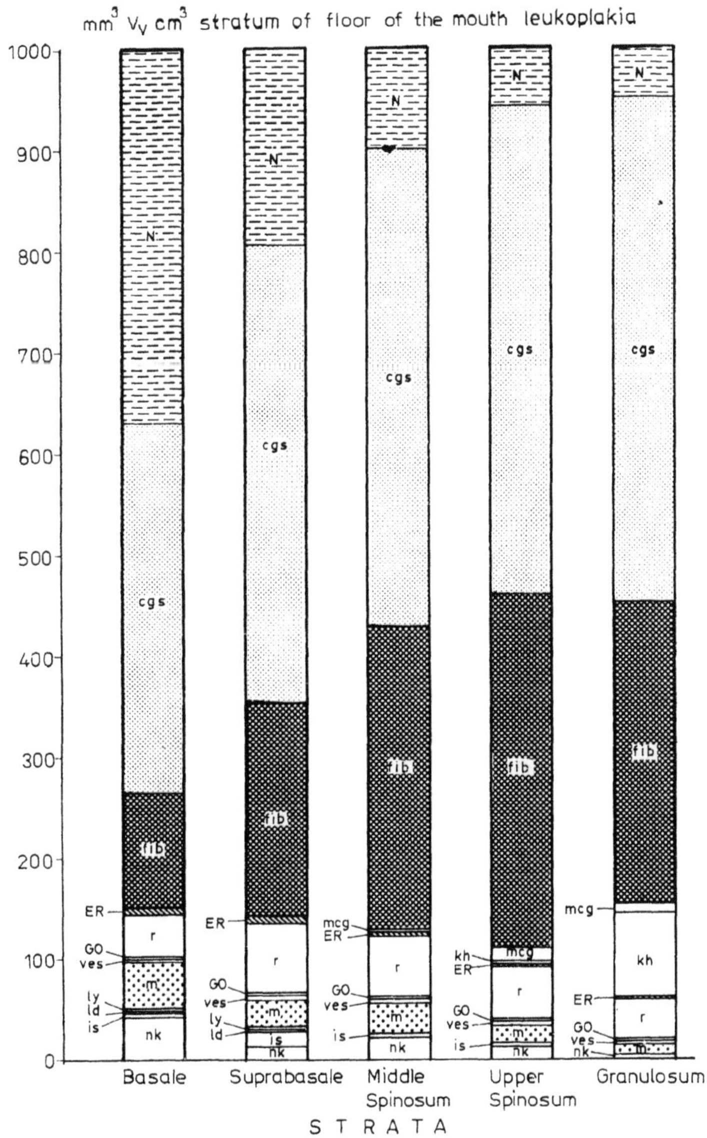

Fig. 87. Diagrammatic presentation of cell components in five layers of epithelial tissue in floor of the mouth leukoplakia (for abbreviations see Fig. 86).

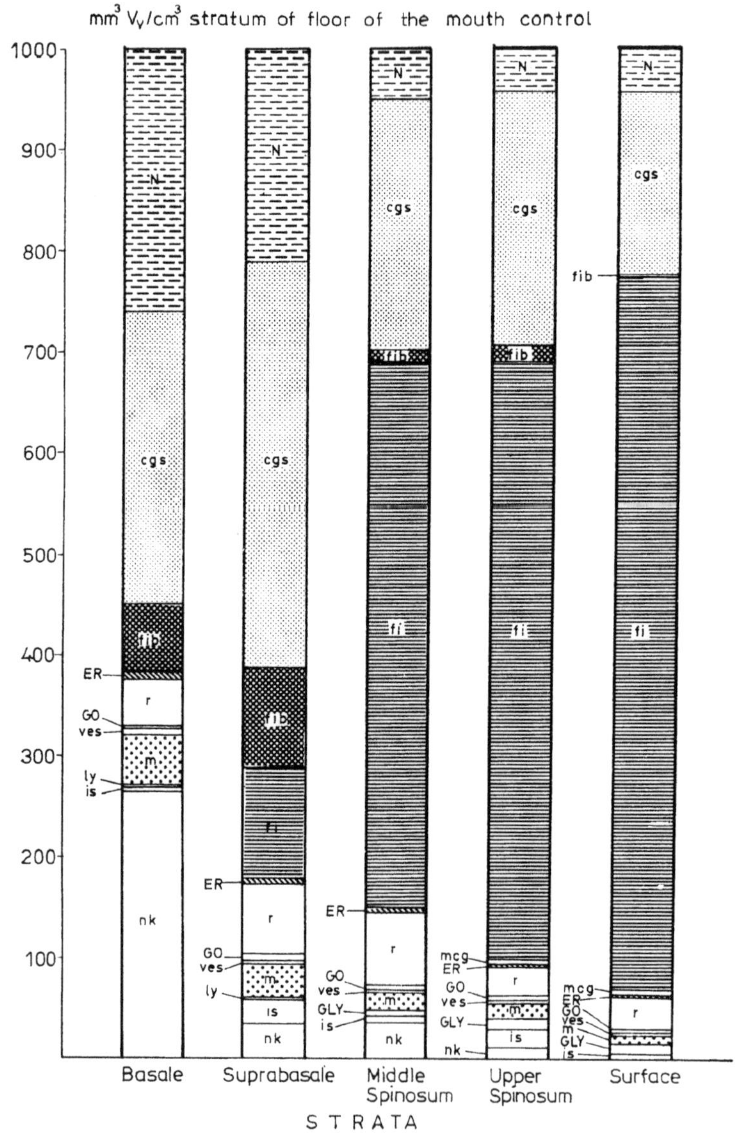

Fig. 88. Diagrammatic presentation of cell components in normal floor of the mouth mucosa, related to the five layers of epithelium examined. fi = single filaments; for other abbreviations see Fig. 86

spinous layers the intercellular spaces were comparatively wider. Desmosome density tended to increase considerably from the basal toward the superficial strata.

Structural density gradients of cytoplasmic organelles

After separating the relatively large nuclear fraction, and the variable non-keratinocyte fraction from each layer, changes in the cytoplasmic components between strata were related to the unit volume of epithelial cytoplasm and were plotted out graphically for evaluation. The volume and surface density gradients had different characteristics in the various epithelia.

The structural gradients of the cytoplasmic components which play a key role in differentiation are shown in Figs 89 and 90.

The volumetric density gradients of cytoplasmic ground substance proved to be identical in the leukoplakic epithelia from both sites and were nearly constant in all strata. The volumetric density of the cytoplasmic ground substance of normal sublingual epithelium was similar to that of keratinizing epithelium in the basal and suprabasal layers, but decreased abruptly in the

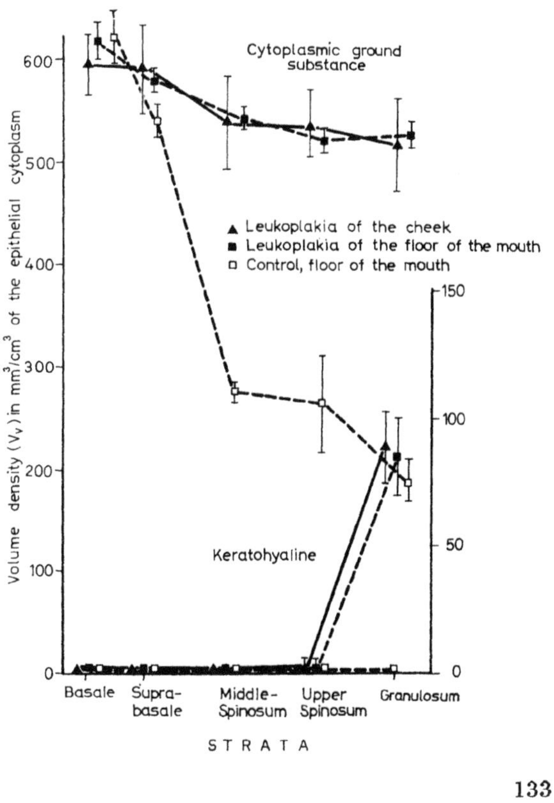

Fig. 89. Characteristic structural gradients of the cytoplasm in normal epithelium. Volume density gradients (in terms of mm^3/cm^3) of cytoplasmic ground substance and keratohyaline granules

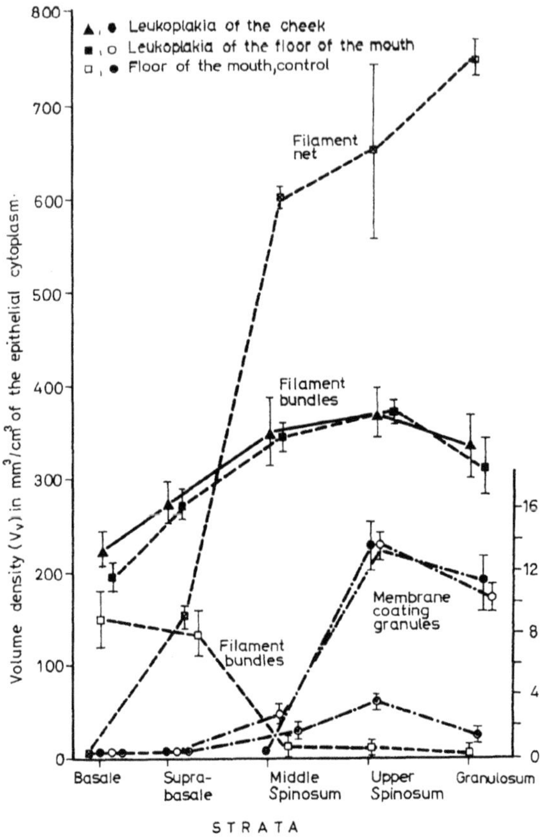

Fig. 90. Characteristic structural gradients of the cytoplasm in leukoplakic oral epithelium. Volume density gradients (in terms of mm^3/cm^3) of cytoplasmic filaments and membrane-coating granules

mid-spinous layer and remained at a low value (25–30%) in the superficial stratum (Fig. 89).

The volumetric density gradients of cytoplasmic filaments were identical in the leukoplakic epithelia of both sites; in these, the filaments occurred exclusively in the form of bundles and occupied 30–35% of the cytoplasm. In contrast, bundled and single filaments occurred in roughly equal proportions in normal sublingual epithelium. The density of the enmeshed single filaments tended to increase toward the superficial layers, where this loose filamentous network filled 60–80% of the cytoplasm. The volumetric fraction of the filament bundles (see Fig. 90) occupied 15% of the cytoplasm in basal and suprabasal cells, but decreased to negligible proportions in the mid-spinous layer and superficial strata.

No keratohyaline granules occurred in the basal, suprabasal and mid-spinous layers of leukoplakic epithelium. The volumetric density of keratohyaline tended to increase gradually above the mid-spinous layer and rose abruptly between the upper spinous and the granular layer. The volumetric density of keratohyaline was identical in the two leukoplakic epithelia, while no keratohyaline granules occurred in normal epithelium (see Fig. 89).

Both leukoplakic epithelia showed a considerable increase in the volumetric fraction of membrane-coating granules between the suprabasal and upper spinous layers, while the normal sublingual epithelium had a low value for this fraction throughout (see Fig. 90).

Morphometry is a relatively new approach to the quantitative characterization of histological parameters (Weibel et al. 1966). Stereological analysis of stratified epithelium was first performed on normal oral mucosa (Schroeder and Münzel-Pedrazzoli 1970, 1973, Meyer and Schroeder 1975, Landay and Schroeder 1976) and later on pathological conditions, such as reticular lichen planus and pemphigoid (Klein–Szántó, et al. 1976, Petrzilka and Schroeder 1976).

All the available information has unequivocally suggested that, through recording quantitative alterations in certain cell components, especially the cytoplasmic organelles, *morphometric analysis can disclose precise information on the differentiation of stratified epithelium.*

In our present study histological and stereological observations have both indicated that leukoplakic lesions of the cheek and floor of the mouth can be regarded as identical because of a similar thickness of epithelium, relative scarcity of connective tissue papillae, and similarities both in histological parameters and in the stereological features of most cytoplasmic components.

Although the epithelial linings of the cheek and floor of the mouth differ in normal conditions (Klein-Szántó and Schroeder 1977) (see Table 47), in the course of keratinization similar changes occur at both sites, resulting in a reduction of epithelial thickness in buccal leukoplakia, but no such alteration in leukoplakia of the floor of the mouth. During keratinization the non-keratinizing epithelium is subject to cornification, analogous to the differentiation of normal epithelium in the hard palate (Meyer and Schroeder 1975). In stereological terms this change involves structural components such as cytoplasmic filaments, membrane-coating granules, keratohyaline granules and cytoplasmic ground substance. This density gradients of the metabolically active organelles (mitochondria, ribosomes, rough surfaced endoplasmic reticulum, Golgi system, etc.) do not differ notably between normal and leukoplakic epithelium. Aggregation of the cytoplasmic filaments into bundles of tonofilament, i.e. an increase in the density of filament bundles, is the most characteristic change associated with both the development of leukoplakia (and the differentiation of normal palatal epithelium) (Meyer and Schroeder 1975). In contrast single filaments form the bulk of the cytoplasmic volume in normal buccal and sublingual epithelium (Fig. 91). It

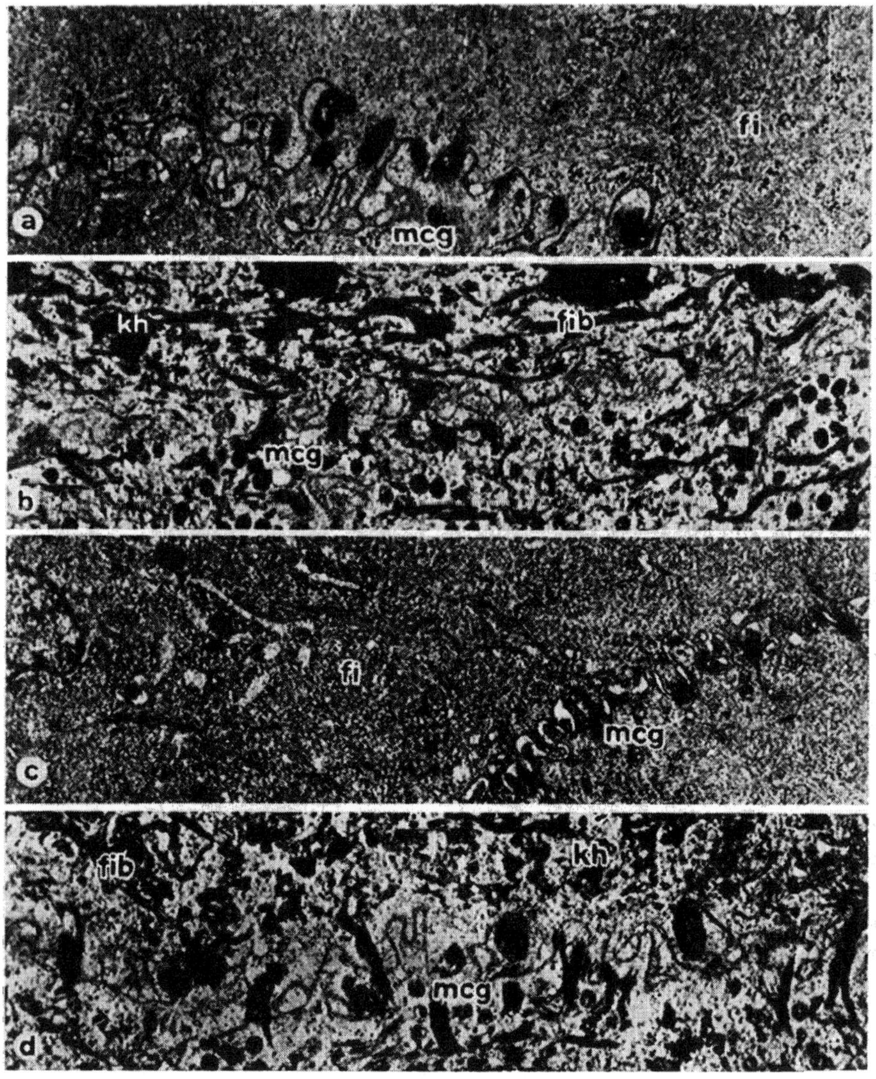

Fig. 91. Electron micrographs of normal and leukoplakic epithelium from the buccal mucosa (*a*, *b*) and floor of the mouth (c, *d*). fi = isolated cytoplasmic filaments constituting a network, fi = filaments aggregated into bundles, mcg = membrane-coating granules, kh = keratohyaline granules. ×40,000

follows that the two groups of simple leukoplakia studied show distinct ultrastructural and architectural differences. In view of these, the lesions can be regarded as metaplastic at the ultrastructural level with an alteration of normal epithelial differentiation.

As to clinical appearance, the simple leukoplakias analyzed for their stereological and histological characteristics were generally sharply delineated homogeneous white lesions (see Figs 83 and 84). In the two cases with pronounced epithelial processes and many connective tissue papillae, not only the stereological data from the lesions, but also their gross appearance differed from the rest. This suggests that there exists within the simple leukoplakias a distinct subgroup with well-defined clinical and histological characteristics. Clinically such lesions appear as homogeneous, solitary white patches with sharply defined outlines and a dry surface, varying in colour from greyish-white to intense white. This particular appearance is a direct result of the special structural features because the colour of the lesion is determined by the actual thickness of the stratum corneum and the degree of epithelial atrophy. According to Payne (1975), keratin formed in leukoplakic epithelium differs chemically from that derived from the normal process of keratinization in oral epithelium (e.g. on the hard palate), and its opaque, whitish colour is due to hydratation of the stratum corneum. Sharply delineated outlines indicate an abrupt transition from normal to leukoplakic epithelium. In such lesions there is usually no inflammatory infiltration of connective tissue.

This type of leukoplakia has been described by many authors (Fasske and Morgenroth 1964, Farman and Lawton 1966, Shafer et al. 1974) who regard it as a clinically defined entity known as simple (L. Sugár and Bánóczy 1969, Bánóczy and Csiba 1972,) or homogeneous leukoplakia (Pindborg 1978). Recently Kramer et al. (1978) have advocated the segregation of sublingual keratosis from the other forms of leukoplakia, on the grounds of its greater tendency to malignant transformation, which is especially associated with lesions that undergo ulceration, develop nodules, or become surrounded by an erythematous halo. There is reason to suppose that some of the lesions of leukoplakia simplex with the clinical features described above might show the histopathological characteristics noted in the present study. Therefore it may be justifiable to regard this type of lesion as a clinically, histopathologically and stereologically well-defined subgroup of oral leukoplakias of the "simple" type.

SCANNING ELECTRON MICROSCOPIC (SEM) EXAMINATIONS

Comparative transmission and scanning electron microscopic studies of human foetal skin and oral mucosa were first performed by Whittaker and Adams (1971). Since then the method has been increasingly employed in the examination of normal and pathological oral mucosa from adults (Svejda and Janota 1974, Schenk and Wersäll 1975, Matsumoto et al. 1976, Svejda et al. 1977, Rudelt and Peters 1978). The scanning electron microscopic examination of oral leukoplakia was initiated by Morgenroth and Morgenroth (1970*a*, *b*, *c*), and continued by Schenk (1975) and Matsumoto et al. (1976). It was established that the delicate surface structure of the superficial epithelial cells assumed a coarse, irregular appearance in leukoplakia, dysplasia or carcinoma, because of the presence of cytoplasmic processes which are also seen in transmission electron micrographs. Of the above authors only Morgenroth and Morgenroth (1970*c*) pursued the correlation between changes seen in the scanning electron microscope and the clinical type of leukoplakia, especially its severe forms which they classified as grades III and IV.

In view of the fact that the differences in the clinical type of leukoplakia are due primarily to dissimilarities in the superficial layers of their epithelium, it seemed worthwhile to examine the scanning electron microscopic features of all clinical types.

We centered our studies on two main aspects; (*i*) whether or not the surface morphology of leukoplakic cells differed between the clinical types, and (*ii*) whether or not the epithelium of dysplastic leukoplakia had similar ultrastructural characteristics to dysplastic lesions of other sites.

Biopsies taken from six patients with leukoplakia of the buccal mucosa were studied together with a specimen of normal buccal mucosa. The group of patients comprised five women and two men, and their age ranged from 42 to 68 years. As to clinical type, of two cases each was either simple, verrucous or erosive leukoplakia. Histological signs of dysplasia were found in one of the two erosive cases. Each specimen of tissue was examined by both transmission and scanning electron microscopy (Bánóczy et al. 1980).

The biopsy specimens were excised with a scalpel under local analgesia (2.5% Lidocaine), washed in isotonic NaCl, fixed in 2.5% glutaraldehyde, washed again in Na-cacodylate buffer (pH 7.4), postfixed in 2% OsO_4, dehydrated in step-graded ethanol, dried in a "Balzers" critical-point drying system, and steam-treated in vacuum (Schaff et al. 1974, Bánóczy et al. (1980).

The surface of normal oral mucosa consisted of a dense, mosaic-like array of polygonal cells which were closely packed. The cell borders were sharply demarcated and the intercellular junctions formed loop-like ridges (Fig. 92).

Fig. 92. Normal buccal mucosa. Polygonal cells in a dense mosaik-like arrangement. Looped prominence represent the intercellular junctions. ×2,880

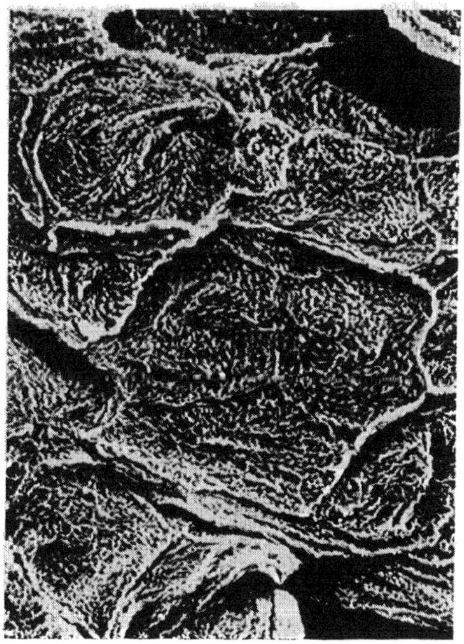

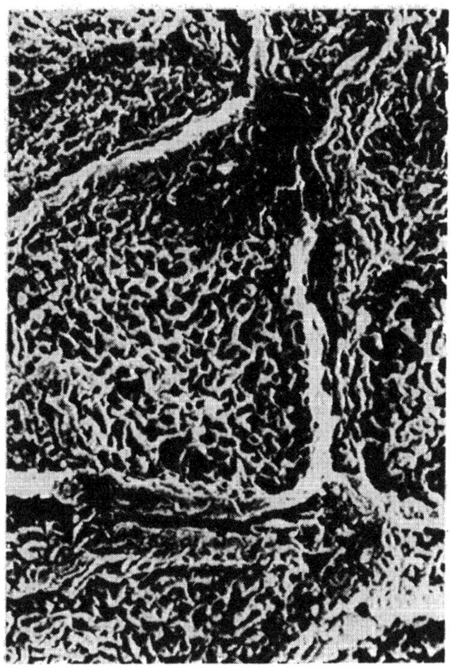

Fig. 93. Normal buccal mucosa. At a higher magnification elevated ridges, the so-called micro-rugae become visible on the cell surface. ×7,200

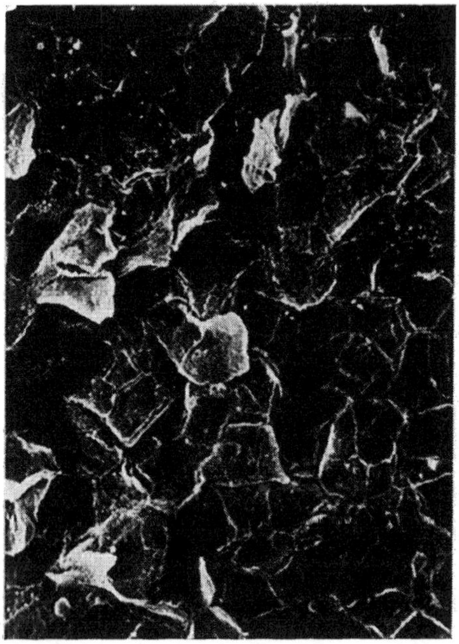

Fig. 94. Simple leukoplakia in a buccal site. Cells arranged in a mosaic-like pattern are for the most part intimately associated with one another, but tend to be drawn apart in places. ×960

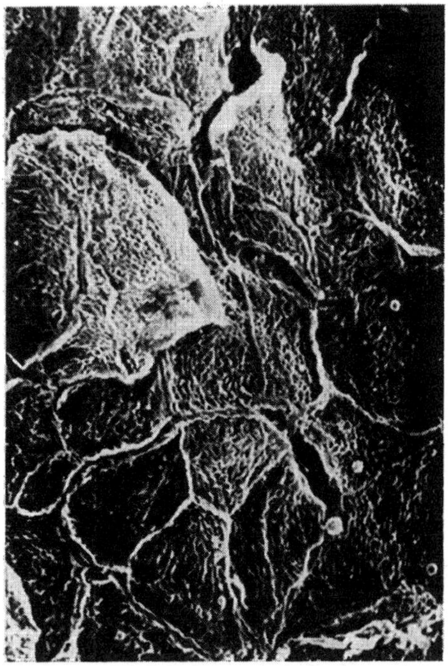

Fig. 95. Simple leukoplakia in a buccal site. The micro-rugal pattern of the cell surfaces is similar to normal. ×2,800

Fig. 96. The same as Fig. 95. ×7,200

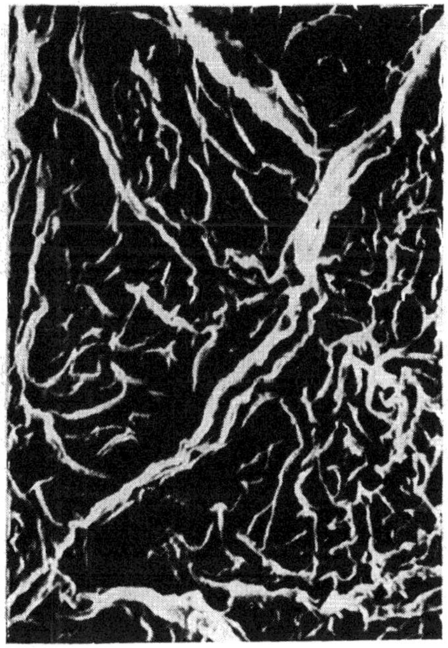

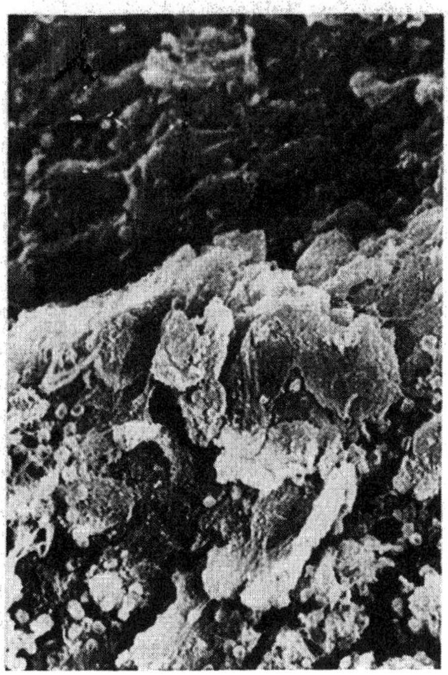

Fig. 97. Verrucous leukoplakia in a buccal site. The superficial layer consists of amorphous, desquamating, hyperkeratotic epithelial cells. ×960

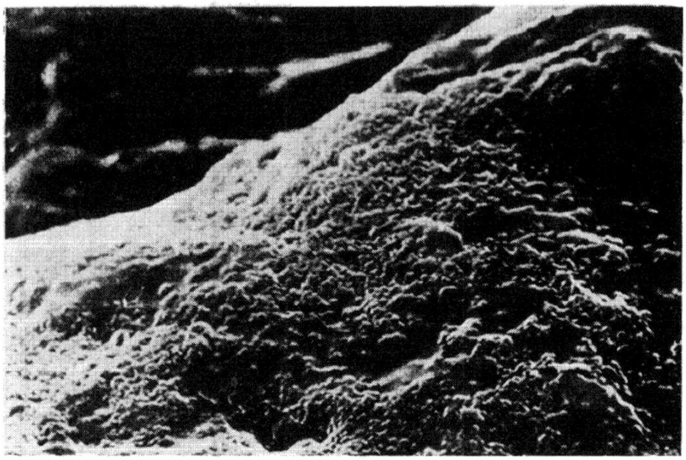

Fig. 98. Verrucous leukoplakia in a buccal site. Only at a higher power of magnification can details of the orderly micro-rugal pattern be seen on the cell surfaces. × 7,360

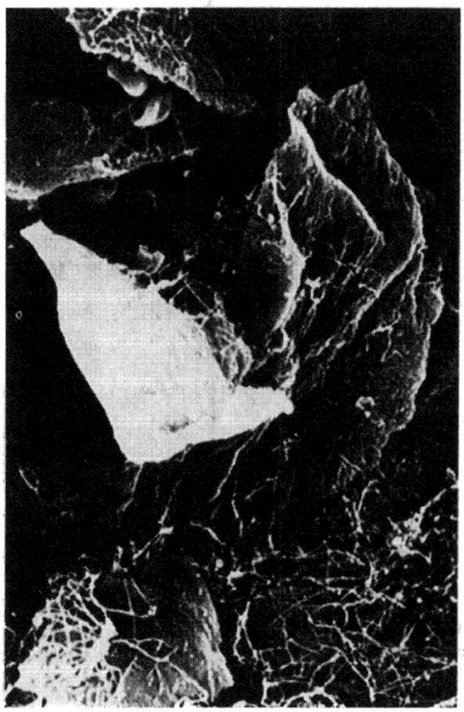

Fig. 99. Erosive leukoplakia in a buccal site. The tight junctions of the epithelial cells have disappeared, leaving empty spaces. The surface is coated by a mass of thread-like micro-organisms. ×7,600

At a higher magnification, parallel rounded, arborizing protrusions (microrugae) formed an orderly pattern on each cell surface (Fig. 93).

In simple leukoplakia, this mosaic-like arrangement of polygonal cells was preserved, but in places some cells overlapped or showed signs of dissociation (Figs 94 and 95). The delicate reticular surface pattern of microrugae was preserved (Fig. 96).

Orthokeratotic thickening of the superficial epithelium (see Fig. 63) is evident grossly and microscopically in verrucous leukoplakia. The scanning electron micrographs showed loss of the polygonal cell outline and of the mosaic-like pattern. The superficial epithelial cells in this hyperkeratosis were shrunken, wrinkled and amorphous, partly desquamated, partly overlapping, and usually with a tight junction at only one pole (Fig. 97). In the high-power micrographs only minor details of the surface pattern preserved (Fig. 98).

The epithelial defects observed grossly and microscopically (see Fig. 75) in erosive leukoplakia were readily seen at the ultrastructural level. The protruding ridges at the intercellular junctions which were seen in epithelium of normal and simple leukoplakia had disappeared altogether. Overlapping cells alternated with large empty spaces, in which solitary hyperkeratotic cells occasionally appeared. The epithelial surface was coated with large masses of predominantly thread-like microorganisms (Fig. 99). Loss of intercellular junctions was also seen at a higher magnification. The surface pattern of the isolated epithelial cells did not show the order seen in normal cells and in simple leukoplakia; the microrugae were irregular and their concentric network was discontinous (Fig. 100). The cytoplasmic invaginations varied in size and thickness, accounting for a disorganized villus pattern at the cell surface (Fig. 101).

Scanning electron microscopy makes possible the three-dimensional study of surfaces with regard to their shape and components (Ohnsorge and Holm 1978). The surface pattern of dysplastic or carcinomatous epithelial cells shows changes which are diagnostically important (Ambrose and Ellison 1968, Jordan and Williams 1971, Schaff et al. 1974, Rubio and Krantz 1976). This observation prompted the use of scanning electron microscopy in studies of the surface of oral precancerous lesions and carcinomas.

Other studies of oral lesions have extended to the interface between oral mucous epithelium and connective tissue (Klein-Szántó and Schroeder 1977), and also to the cytoplasmic processes of basal cells (Schenk 1975). Dysplastic basal cells had marked irregularities in the shape and arrangement of cytoplasmic processes compared normal.

Schenk (1975) saw a special advantage in scanning electron microscopy since it enables the study of the very layers that are usually inaccessible to transmission electron microscopy because they are destroyed by processing,

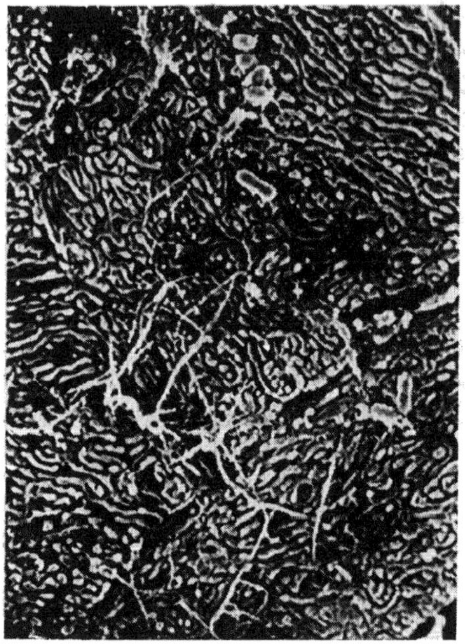

Fig. 100. Erosive leukoplakia in a buccal site. The micro-rugal pattern is irregular and discontinuous in places. ×960

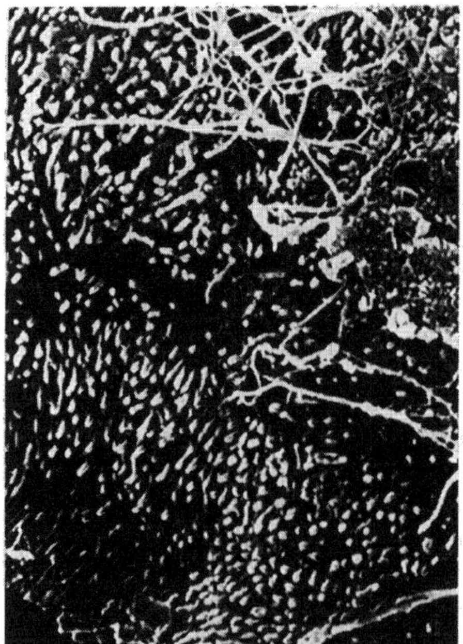

Fig. 101. Erosive leukoplakia in a buccal site. Note cytoplasmic invaginations of various shapes and sizes, and the villus-like surface pattern. ×9,600

e.g. the stratum corneum. Conversely, the value of scanning electron microscopy in the study of precancerosis and leukoplakia might be disputed, as is the value of exfoliative cytology, on the grounds that in some leukoplakias hyperkeratosis may mask dysplastic changes in more deeply-seated cells.

In the cases studied by us, *scanning electron micrographs made possible the differentiation between superficial epithelial cells of normal mucosa and leukoplakia, and between the different clinical types of leukoplakia.*

In simple leukoplakia, presentation of continuity in the superficial cell layer, the morphology of intercellular junctions, and the microrugal surface pattern of the cells was in every respect similar to normal oral epithelium, except for the presence of a few desquamating, keratinized cells. In verrucous leukoplakia the surface layer consisted of characteristically shrunken, desquamated, hyperkeratotic cells with a defective surface pattern. Superficial hyperkeratosis presumably prevents cells from the deeper layers, from emerging onto the surface for evaluation, as already implied from cytological studies (Silverman 1959, Silverman et al. 1958, Umiker et al. 1960, Gardner 1964, Bánóczy and Rigó 1976). However, erosive leukoplakia had a discontinuous, superficial layer and an abnormal, pleomorphic cell surface pattern. The villus-like pattern found in one of the two dysplastic cases was in all probability formed by free desmosomes or cytoplasmic processes, which had become detached after disruption of the intercellular junctions.

Several authors (Schaff et al. 1974, Schenk 1975, Matsumoto et al. 1976) agree that the main value of scanning electron microscopy is in the detection of changes in the size and arrangement of the superficial cytoplasmic processes which are also seen by transmission electron microscopy. This application of the scanning technique has been used in the study of malignant or premalignant changes in other epithelia such as those of the uterine cervix, urinary bladder, and lung (Rubio and Krantz 1976, Jacobs et al. 1976, Takenaga et al. 1977). In line with observations made on other epithelia we found in a dysplastic lesion of erosive leukoplakia an obviously abnormal, pleomorphic arrangement of the cytoplasmic processes. This indicates that the scanning technique may supply important new information about the distinctly precancerous forms of erosive leukoplakia.

CHAPTER VII

ORAL "WHITE LESIONS" OTHER THAN LEUKOPLAKIA

Expansion of knowledge and improvement in diagnostic procedures have permitted discrimination between certain lesions which grossly resemble leukoplakia, and which collectively are termed "white lesions" in the Anglo-Saxon literature. These clinico-pathological entities include lichen planus, leukoedema exfoliativum mucosae oris (white sponge naevus) and morsicatio buccarum et labiorum.

Patients seen in the Clinic of Maxillo-Facial Surgery and Dentistry, Dental Faculty of Semmelweis University Medical School, Budapest with these white lesions were also included in our follow-up studies in order to obtain more information on their clinical and pathological aspects, therapy, diagnostic differentiation, and liability to malignant transformation.

CLINICAL (LONGITUDINAL) STUDIES OF PATIENTS WITH ORAL LICHEN PLANUS

The oral signs of lichen planus frequently cause diagnostic problems for dentists. The lesion occasionally arouses the suspicion of cancer not only in the patient but also in the clinician. As the etiology of the condition is still unknown, specific therapy is problematical, while empirical treatment may often fail, or the lesion may heal spontaneously. Reports of a rising incidence of malignant change in oral lichen planus during the recent years have prompted the investigators to attach increasing importance to the disease.

The frequency of occurrence of oral lichen planus has been little studied. Hazen (1935) gave its prevalence among American Negroes as 0.29%. Mehta et al. (1971) found an 0.1% prevalence in rural Indian communities, while in the Kerala province of India Pindborg et al. (1972) found a prevalence of 1.5%.

In Hungary, Bánóczy et al. (1969) found oral lichen planus in 0.6% of 16,332 persons in a stomato-oncological screening programme. Among dental patients in India, Pindborg et al. (1966) found the lesion in 0.02–0.22% of subjects, while Lauffer and Kuffer (1970) in 0.44, 0.58, %, Shklar (1972) in 0.5%, and Wilsch et al. (1978) in 0.63%, respectively. In Sweden, Axell (1975) observed an 1.6% prevalence of oral lichen in an unselected population. Among all dental outpatients seen in the Clinic of Maxillo-Facial Surgery and Dentistry, Dental Faculty of Semmelweis University Medical School, Budapest, from 1965 to 1970, 0.39% had oral lichen planus.

In the period from 1954 to 1975, several authors reported comprehensive studies of groups of patients with oral lichen planus (Cooke 1954, Simpson 1957, Dechaume et al. 1957, Warin et al. 1958, Shklar and McCarthy 1961, Hermann 1963, Andreasen 1968*a, b,* Dechaume and Payen 1969, Silverman and Griffith 1974). The largest groups, numbering 600, 327, 213 and 611 patients, were surveyed by Shklar (1972), Fulling (1973), McClatchey et al. (1975), and Neumann-Jensen et al. (1977), respectively.

Opinions have been divergent as to whether or not oral lichen planus is precancerous. Cancer development from oral lichen was first reported by Hallopeau (1910). According to Lauffer and Kuffer (1970), a total of 90 cases of a carcinomatous change in lichen oris had been reported in the world literature up to 1970. Since then Kuffer and his colleagues (1975) have described another 40 cases (Cernéa et al. 1971*a, b*) bringing the total of reported cases to about 150. The frequency of cancer development in oral lichen planus had been estimated by different authors to be up to 10% (Lauffer and Kuffer 1970).

In the Clinic of Maxillo-Facial Surgery and Dentistry, Dental Faculty of Semmelweis University Medical School, Budapest, 326 patients were diagnosed as having oral lichen planus between 1960 and 1969. An evaluation of these cases has been described in detail (Kövesi and Bánóczy 1973*a, b, c.*) We made a clinical diagnosis of lichen planus if the lesion had the characteristic Wickham's striae. Some of these lesions were also examined histologically. The typical microscopic appearance of lichen oris were recognized as hyperkeratosis, hydropic and vacuolar degeneration of the basal layer, bandlike infiltration of round cells, and an eosinophilic acellular layer in the connective tissue (Andreasen 1968*b*, Kramer et al. 1970*a, b,* McClatchey et al. 1975).

Examination of the *age and sex distribution* of lichen oris showed a nearly equal incidence in the age groups 40–69 of the female sex, but a prevalence of men in the range 50 and 59 years. *Overall 62.6% of our patients were women* (Table 48).

The actual prevalence of lichen oris among our patients is compared in Table 49 with the calculated prevalence based on the census returns for 1960 and 1970 (Statisztikai Évkönyv 1960, 1970).

Oral lichen usually occurred in subjects over 40 years of age (86.5%), and was especially frequent between 50 and 59 years. Calculations based on population statistics indicated that it is not as rare above 70 years of age as

Table 48

Age and sex distribution of patients with oral lichen

Age (years)	Men		Women		Total	
	No.	%	No.	%	No.	%
20–29	4	3.3	3	1.5	7	2.1
30–39	14	11.5	23	11.3	37	11.3
40–49	21	17.2	53	26.0	74	22.7
50–59	37	30.3	55	27.0	92	28.2
60–69	30	24.6	54	26.4	84	25.8
>70	16	13.1	16	7.8	32	9.9
Totals	122	100.0	204	100.0	326	100.0

Table 49

Computed and actual age group distribution of patients with oral lichen (males + females)

Age (years)	Computed	Actual	Actual / Computed
20–29	68.49	7	0.10
30–39	67.79	37	0.55
40–49	61.76	74	1.20
50–59	54.53	92	1.69
60–69	44.12	84	1.90
>70	29.31	32	1.09
Totals	326.00	326	

Table 50

Frequency of different etiological factors in lichen oris

Etiological factors	Cases	
	No.	%
Smoking habit	48	14.7
Electric potential difference	47	14.4
Dental inflammatory focus	67	20.3
Psychological factors	73	22.3
Other factors	129	39.5

(In some cases several causal factors were simultaneously present.)

suggested by the actual number of such cases (which was less than one-third of the number in the 50–59-year-old age group).

Analysis of the *case histories* showed that oral lichen caused symptoms in the great majority (90.7%) of the cases, and in the few instances (9.3%) when it did not, the lesion was not noticed by the patient but only by the dentist.

Of the possible *etiological factors* we examined those most frequently incriminated by other authors and by the patients themselves. As shown in Table 50, smoking, electric potential difference (Fig. 102), dental inflammatory foci and psychological factors were present in roughly equal proportions (14.4–22.3%). As to other factors of the 129 patients 17 (13.9%) were diabetics, chronic mechanical irritation was found in 13.9% of the cases, and anaemia in 13.1% (see Table 50).

The clinical types of oral lichen have been variously classified by other authors into 8 to 10 groups. We recognized six types; papular (Fig. 102), reticular (colour photo 11), plaque-like (Fig. 103), bullous (Fig. 104), atrophic (colour photo 12) and erosive (colour photo 13), in relation to the criteria established by Andreasen (1968*a*).

As to the occurrence of each type, in our patients *reticular type was most prevalent* (168 cases; 51.5%), *followed by the erosive* (90 cases; 27.6%), atrophic and papular (41 cases; 12.6%), and bullous type (27 cases; 8.3%) (Table 51).

The overall frequency of concurrent cutaneous lesions was 19.3% (Table 51), *and the frequency in relation with the clinical type was lower in the reticular and erosive forms* (17.4 and 15.5%) than in the papular–atrophic

Table 51

Occurrence of cutaneous symptoms with the different clinical types of oral lichen

Clinical type	No. of cases	Cases showing cutaneous symptoms	
		No.	%
Reticular	168	29	17.4
Papular	13	3	29.3 (Papular, Plaque, Atrophic combined)
Plaque	12	3	
Atrophic	16	6	
Bullous	27	8	29.6
Erosive	90	14	15.5
Totals	326	63	19.3

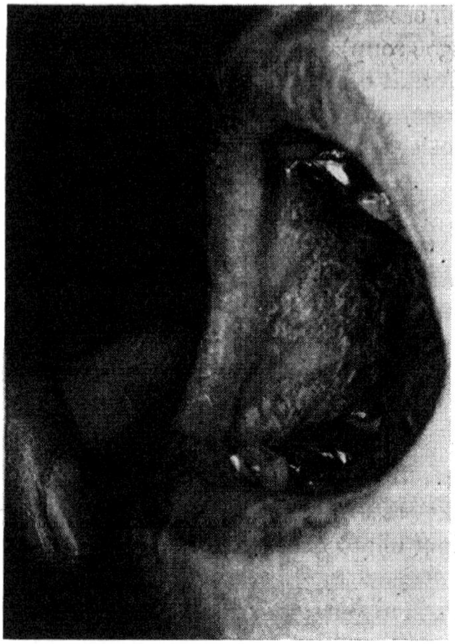

Fig. 102. Papular lichen in the buccal n.u cosa of a 52-year-old female patient. The papular lesions are solitary or confluent. A high electric potential difference was demonstrated between metal restorations

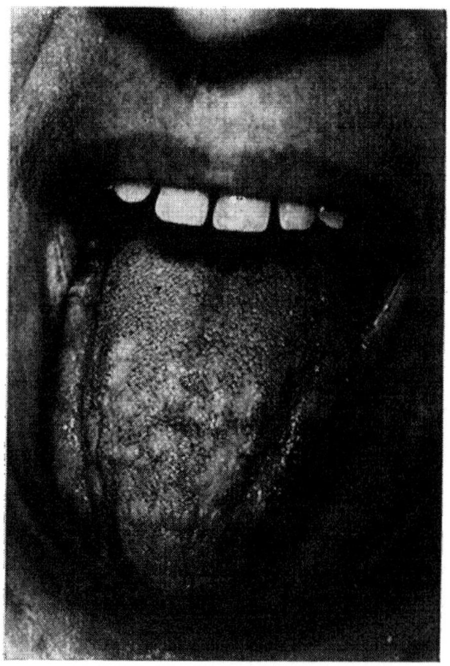

Fig. 103. Plaque-like confluence of lichen oris papillae on the tongue of a 73-year-old female patient

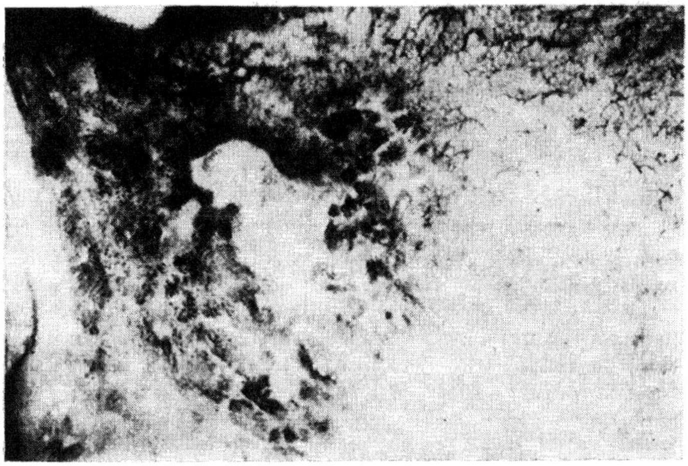

Fig. 104. Bullons lichen at the border between the hard and soft palates of an 52-year-old male patient. The lesion is surrounded by a hyperaemic zone with the characteristic striae of Wickham

and bullous ones (29.3 and 29.6%), but this difference was not statistically significant.

The follow-up periods for oral lichen are shown in Table 52. Of the 326 patients, 274 (84%) presented for re-examination, and 53 did not. The average length of observation was 3 years for the 274 patients.

Treatment, apart from the restoration of oral hygiene, included vitamin A and B or steroid therapy and surgical removal. The results are shown in Table 53.

Table 52

Periods of observation in cases of lichen oris

Period of observation (years)	Cases	
	No.	%
<1	134	41.4
>1–<5	101	30.0
>5–<10	35	11.0
Patients not available for control	52	16.1
Totals	326	100.0

Table 53

Methods and results of treatment

Method of treatment \ Result	Healed		Improved		Unchanged		Improvement followed by relapse		Total	
	No.	%	No.	%	No.	%	No.	%	No.	%
Restoration of oral hygiene without any other treatment	7	20.6	21	61.8	6	17.6	—	—	34	100
Vitamin A and B therapy	25	13.6	114	62.0	28	15.2	17	9.2	184	100
Steroid treatment	4	9.5	19	45.2	8	19.1	11	26.2	42	100
Surgical treatment	7	53.8	3	23.1	3	23.1	—	—	13	100
Totals	43	15.7	157	57.5	45	16.5	28	10.3	273	100

Restoration of oral hygiene, i.e. removal of teeth with septic foci and of inadequate metal restorations, and/or the exchange of restorations giving rise to electric potential differences, was followed by healing or improvement of the lesion in seven (20.6 %) and 21 (61.8 %) of such cases, respectively, but had no effect in six cases (17.6 %). In the remaining 184 cases dental treatment was combined with other therapeutic measures, so that its independent evaluation was not possible.

Local or parenteral administration of vitamins A and B was given for two to three months. The lesion healed or improved in 25 (13.6 %) and 114 (62.0 %) of the 184 cases, respectively, and failed to improve in 28 cases (15.2 %), and initial improvement was followed by relapse after vitamin withdrawal in 17 cases (9.2 %).

Steroids were given in the form of Prednisolone tablets, in repeated courses of decreasing dosage for periods of 1–2 weeks, separated by intervals without medication. Of the 42 patients so treated, four (9.5 %), 19 (45.2 %) and eight (19.1 %) showed healing, improvement and no change, respectively, while 11 patients (26.2 %) relapsed on withdrawal of the drug after a temporary improvement.

In view of the good results obtained by Gombos et al. (1973) from the use of tranquilizers, we attempted such sedation in cases where the etiological role of mental stress was suspected. However, the patients were unresponsive to this therapeutic approach, and such drugs were later used only as adjuvants to other forms of treatment.

There was surgical intervention in 13 cases with long-standing, small and usually erosive lesions, refractory to all other treatments. Surgical excision was followed by complete healing in seven cases (53.8 %) and by improvement in three cases, but it was ineffective in the other three.

Of the 274 cases of oral lichen in our follow-up study only one (0.4 %) showed a carcinomatous change. This case is described in detail by Sallay and Csiba (1973); the carcinoma developed in an erosive type of lichen on the tongue of an aged female, who had been examined regularly.

On examining the age and sex distribution of oral lichen planus, Schmidt (1961) and Depaoli (1964) found it most prevalent between 30 and 60 years of age, with a slight shift towards a higher age incidence in females. Data from dermatological and stomatological statistics give the percentage incidence in women as 53.8 and 56.2 %, respectively. Our findings are similar to those of other authors except Mehta et al. (1971), who found a male to female ratio of 2.2:1 in India.

The importance of various etiological factors was assessed in comparison to their possible role in the etiology of oral leukoplakia. In Hungary the proportion of smokers is about 50 % in the total population and about 83 % among patients with oral leukoplakia (L. Sugár and Bánóczy 1970). Bearing in mind the fact that 46 % of patients with oral lichen seen by Neumann-Jensen and co-workers (1977) were smokers, the 14.4 % smokers found by us is a very low incidence. In contrast the etiological significance of electric potential difference (14.4 %) was increased several times over that found in oral leukoplakia (3 %) (Bánóczy and L. Sugár 1972). This indicates the major etiological importance of bioelectrics in oral lichen, as emphasized by Frykholm et al. (1969) and ourselves (Inovay and Bánóczy 1960*a*, *b*, 1961, Bánóczy et al. 1979).

Our suggestion that diabetes may predispose to oral lichen planus, correlates well with the observation of Grinspan et al. (1966) that among 110 diabetic patients 37.7 % had also suffered from lichen. We also agree with other authors about the importance of dental foci, and psychological factors. In addition, recent stereological–morphometric investigations (Klein-Szántó et al. 1976) have suggested the etiological involvement of autoimmune mechanisms in oral lichen.

As to the distribution of clinical types, Neumann-Jensen et al. (1977) agreed with us that the reticular type is prevalent, but they found a considerably greater incidence of the plaque and atrophic types.

The incidence of cutaneous lesions varies significantly when estimated by either stomatologists or dermatologists. The figures given by stomatologists are wide-varying; i.e. Konstantinov et al. (1959) 4–5 %, Grinspan et al. (1966) 25 %, Renstrup and Pindborg (1958) 33 %, Andreasen (1968*a*) 44 %. On the basis of our own experience we agree with Andreasen (1968*a*) that cutaneous symptoms are less frequently associated with erosive oral lichen than with other types.

The proportion of patients available for follow-up study was greater (84%) for oral lichen than for leukoplakia (72.3%) (Bánóczy and L. Sugár 1972). Patients with lichen presented for re-examination willingly, probably due to the psychological factors mentioned earlier.

Among the possible treatments vitamin therapy was greatly preferred because of its safety, but it gave equivocal results. Andreasen (1968*a*) reported partial remissions during treatment with vitamin A.

Steroids have been widely used in the treatment of lichen oris during the last 20 years. In comparative studies with arsenic, mercury and steroid medication Samman (1956) found a lasting improvement only in the group treated with steroids. Fülöp (1957) reported efficient treatment of the cutaneous symptoms of lichen planus with ACTH. Mumford and Morgan (1956) observed a rapid exacerbation of the disease after withdrawal of cortisone and ACTH, and Andreasen (1968*a*) made similar observations. Sallay (1969) obtained good results with the intra-lesional injection of microcrystals, and Kövesi (1973) with treatment with chloroquine.

Surgical removal of lichen planus is rarely attempted. Schettler and Koberg (1970) thought biopsy and surgical intervention indispensable in cases suspected of malignant transformation. This justifies our successful surgical intervention in cases with small, long-standing erosive areas of lichen oris.

The finding of only a single case of malignant transformation (0.4%) in our large group of patients failes to substantiate the view that lichen oris is precancerous. Shklar (1972), Fulling (1973) and Khrutchkoff et al. (1978) hold the view that the concurrence of lichen and carcinoma is a mere coincidence, while other authors (Andreasen and Pindborg 1963, Schettler and Koberg 1970, Sallay and Csiba 1973, Kövesi et al. 1975) regard oral lichen as a frankly precancerous lesion.

Silverman and Griffith (1974) concluded that since the incidence of cancer was considerably greater (2.5%) in their group of patients with oral lichen than in a control population (0.05%), the risk of oral cancer may be increased in the presence of lichen oris. According to Lauffer and Kuffer (1970), cancer develops from oral lichen much more frequently than is reported; they, too, held the view that lichen oris is precancerous condition. Two factors have been believed to be of a major importance in the malignant transformation of oral lichen: (*i*) the vulnerability of the oral mucosa after frequent exacerbations of the lesion, which may predispose to erosive change and tumour formation (Kuffer 1972, Sonkodi and Boda 1977) and (*ii*) the duration of the lesion, since it is usually lesions which have been present for one or more decades that become malignant (Kuffer 1975). The single case of cancer development in our follow-up study of oral lichen and another *carcinoma in lichen planus* observed by us earlier (L. Sugár and Bánóczy 1957, 1959), both *arose from erosive lichen, which indicates that this clinical type may be susceptible to malignant change.* It should be noted that the observation period was much shorter in our cases than in Kuffer's (1975); this would probably account for the lower incidence of malignant change found by us.

SIMULTANEOUS OCCURRENCE OF LEUKOPLAKIA AND ORAL LICHEN

Although clinical and histological diagnostic criteria for leukoplakia and lichen oris are well-established, differentiation of the two conditions may still be problematical to both the clinician and the histopathologist. The possibility of the simultaneous occurrence of the two lesions cannot always be excluded (Shklar 1972). As far as we know, co-existence of the two conditions has been reported only once (McClatchey et al. 1975). We therefore selected from the 520 cases of leukoplakia and 326 cases of lichen oris those which had both lesions either simultaneously or in succession, in order to clarify whether

— leukoplakia and lichen oris often occur simultaneously, or transform into one another,

and

— whether the co-existence of the two conditions is of clinical significance (Bánóczy et al. 1979).

Of the total of 864 patients, 27 (3.2%) had both lesions through a mean observation period of 5.8 years.

Table 54 shows the age and sex distribution of the patients affected by both lesions. Of the 27 patients, 18 were over 40 years of age.

Table 54

Age and sex distribution of patients simultaneously affected by leukoplakia and lichen oris

Age (years)	Men	Women	Totals
<30	2	—	2
30–39	3	4	7
40–49	4	2	6
50–59	1	5	6
60–69	2	3	5
>70	—	1	1
Totals	12	15	27

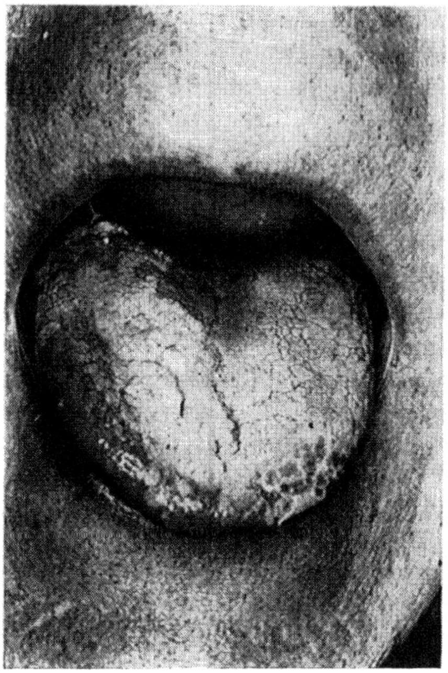

Fig. 105. Co-existent verrucous leukoplakia and reticular lichen on the tongue of a 72-year-old male patient

Clinically erosive leukoplakia was most common among the patients with both conditions (Table 55). The lichen lesions were reticular, plaque, or erosive in type; no papular, bullous or atrophic lesions were found. Combination of the two lesions was more frequent in identical than non-identical grades of severity (Fig 105).

Table 56 shows the site distribution in percentage terms. It should be noted that several oral regions were involved in some cases. The most frequent

Table 55

Clinical type distribution of co-existent leukoplakia and lichen oris

Lichen \ Leukoplakia	Simplex	Verrucous	Erosive	Total
Reticular	8	5	3	16
Plaque	—	3	2	5
Erosive	—	—	6	6
Totals	8	8	11	27

Table 56

Site distribution of co-existent oral leukoplakia and lichen

Localization	Percentage occurrence %
Buccal mucosa	51.4
Tongue	21.6
Lips	8.1
Commissures	8.1
Hard palate	2.7
Soft palate	2.7
Floor of the mouth	5.4
Totals	100.0

sites of leukoplakia and lichen were the buccal mucosa and the tongue (Fig. 105).

Examination for variations in the site and time of occurrence showed that leukoplakia and lichen occurred

in the same site at the same time (Fig. 105)	in 6 cases
in the same site at different times (Fig. 108)	in 16 cases
in different sites at the same time	in 4 cases
in different sites at different times	in 1 case
	27 cases

Table 57 shows the therapeutic results in relation to the initial or major clinical diagnosis. It should be noted that in three cases of lichen oris, leukoplakia developed after a chloroquine treatment.

Table 57

Therapeutic results in co-existent lichen and leukoplakia

Clinical diagnosis \ Treatment	Healed	Improved	Unchanged	Worse	Carcinoma	Totals
Lichen oris	1	6	4	1	1	13
Leukoplakia	2	8	3	—	1	14
Totals	3	14	4	1	2	27

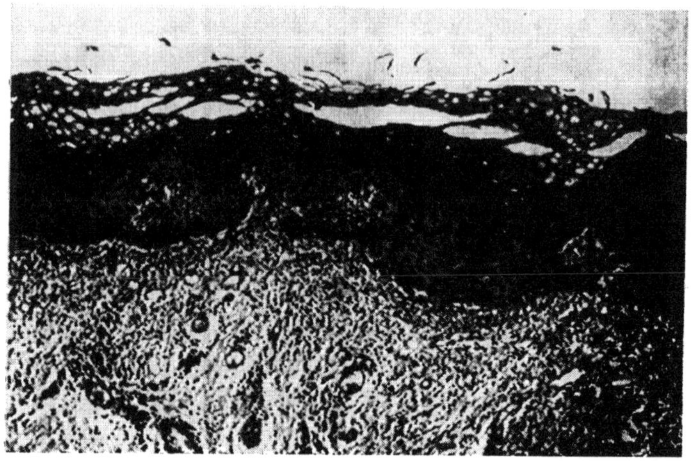

Fig. 106. Light micrograph of a biopsy from the leukoplakia shown in Fig. 105. The thickness of the epithelium is normal, hyperorthokeratosis is present with a distinct stratum granulosum, and the connective tissue shows a moderately severe inflammatory cell reaction. H. & E., ×125

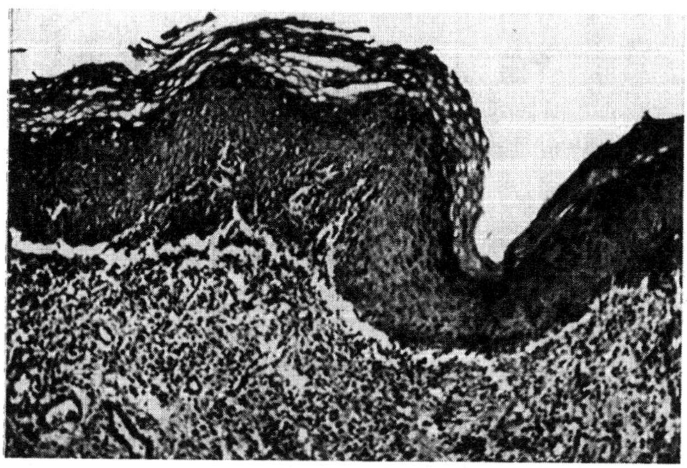

Fig. 107. Light micrograph of a biopsy from the lichenoid lesion shown in Fig. 105. Some parts are acanthotic, there is hyperortho- and hyperparakeratosis with a stratum granulosum, a gap has formed between epithelial and connective tissue, and the latter is densely infiltrated by lymphocytes. H. & E., ×125

Among the 27 cases of co-existent leukoplakia and lichen, one or more biopsies were taken from 17. A total 32 biopsy specimens were available for histological examination.

The main histological changes are listed below:

a. hyperkeratosis with stratum granulosum
b. acanthosis
c. oedema of the spinous layer
d. vacuolar degeneration of the basal layer
e. separation of epithelium from connective tissue (subepithelial bulla)
f. appearance of an acellular eosinophilic band underneath the basement membrane
g. band-like lymphocitic infiltration in the connective tissue
h. dyskeratosis

Of the above changes (d), (e) and (f) were found to be of value as differentiating features (Fig. 107), for none of them occurred in clinically identified cases of leukoplakia, while one or two, most frequently all three, were always present in lichen oris. Most of the lichen cases had unusually large and dark-staining keratohyaline granules, interspersed throughout the stratum spinosum.

Analysis of the clinical and histological features in relation to time and site, led to the following conclusions:

a. Of the 17 biopsies, 4 showed the joint occurrence of leukoplakia and lichen, by clinical and histological criteria, at the same time and in the same place. The microscopic appearance of the lesion was characteristic of lichen oris, but also had some of the non-specific changes associated with leukoplakia (Figs 105—107).
b. The clinical and histological diagnosis were at variance in six cases. In three of these classified as leukoplakia, there was the microscopic appearance of lichen oris, while in the other three, diagnosed clinically as lichen, there was non-specific keratosis on histological examination.
c. Two patients showed changes in both the clinical and histological characteristics of lesions located at the same site, during the period of observation (Figs 108–110). In these cases transformation of one lesion into the other clearly occurred.

Epithelial dysplasia was found in eight cases; cancer developed in two cases, after the disease had existed for 20 and 30 years.

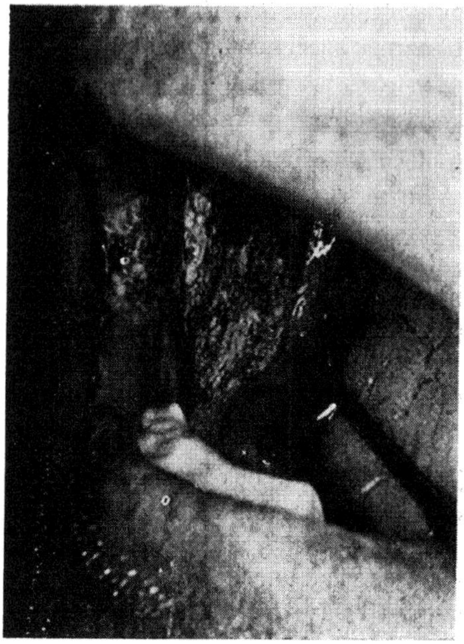

Fig. 108. Erosive leukoplakia with histological indications of a severe dysplasia in the buccal mucosa of a 60-year-old male patient. Twenty years earlier histologically verified lichen developed in the same site

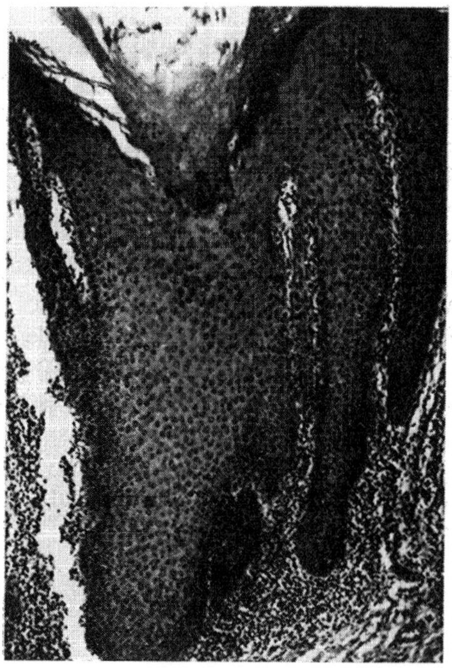

Fig. 109. Light micrograph of a biopsy taken twenty years ago, from the buccal mucosa shown in Fig. 108 which had the clinical appearance of lichen planus. Note epithelial hyperplasia, acanthosis, hyperparakeratosis, separation of epithelium and connective tissue, and a band-like infiltration of lymphocytes. H. & E., ×125

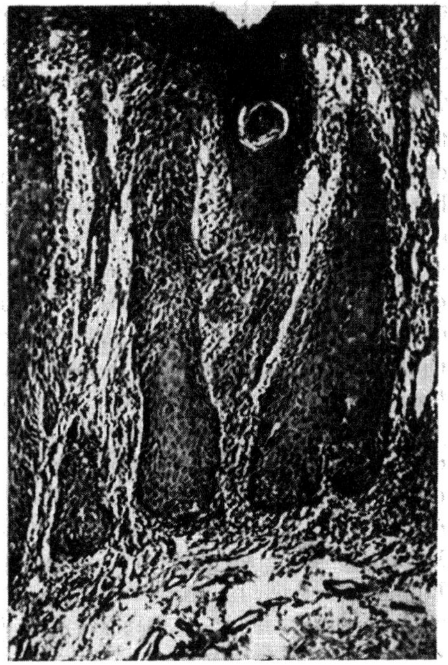

Fig. 110. Microscopic appearance of the erosive buccal leukoplakia shown in Fig. 108. Epithelial hyperplasia, finger-like epithelial ridges, irregular stratification of the epithelium, hyperplasia and loss of polarity of basal cells, dyskeratosis, splitting of intercellular junctions, alteration of the nuclear : cytoplasmic ratio, cellular polymorphism. H. & E., ×125

McClatchey and co-workers (1975) found co-existence with leukoplakia in seven (3.5%) of 200 cases of lichen oris, a similar frequency to our 3.2%. The age and sex distribution corresponded to that observed in our total groups of lichen and leukoplakia (Bánóczy and L. Sugár 1972, Kövesi and Bánóczy 1973*a*, *b*).

Erosive leukoplakia was the lesion most often co-existent with lichen planus. Our previous observation (Bánóczy and L. Sugár 1975) that erosive leukoplakia is the most changeable of all types is in part substantiated by this observation.

The plaque type of lichen, which occurred in 18.5% of our cases, was observed by Neumann-Jensen and co-workers (1977) to develop from reticular or atrophic lesions in smokers. In view of this, they thought it possible that superimposition of leukoplakia upon lichen was influenced by smoking.

Of the various clinical types of lichen, papular, bullous and atrophic lesions were not encountered in this material. Kuffer (1972) believes that atrophic lichen is a persistent condition and this might account for its reduced potential to transform to other types. In our experience, co-existent lesions were chiefly combinations of either slight or severe grades of the two conditions: erosive leukoplakia and erosive lichen were co-existent in 22.2% of the cases, simple leukoplakia and reticular lichen in 29.6%, while combinations of mixed grade were less frequent (see Table 55).

The most common sites of co-existent lesions were the cheek and tongue. The loose structure of the oral mucosa in these regions may be related to an increased rate of cell turnover, which in turn could account for a greater liability to change of any kind. Changes in the clinical type of oral leukoplakia, described in a previous chapter, were also most frequent in these sites (Bánóczy and L. Sugár 1975).

Lesions of oral lichen which gave rise to superimposed leukoplakia after chloroquine medication were originally of erosive type. Healing of the erosion may have involved hyperkeratosis which would account for the clinical appearance of leukoplakia. Induced hyperkeratosis may also occur from the influence of smoking (Neumann-Jensen et al. 1977).

We identified lichen both clinically and histologically, but leukoplakia only clinically in our studies of co-existent lesions. The main histological characteristics of lichen were vacuolar degeneration of the basal cells, presence of an acellular eosinophilic zone beneath the epithelium and subepithelial bulla formation. As hyperkeratosis occurred equally in lichen and leukoplakia, it had no value as a discriminant feature.

Shklar and Meyer (1961) gave the diagnostic criteria of lichen at the microscopic level as para- and/or hyperkeratosis, hydropic degeneration of the stratum germinativum and a band-like chronic inflammatory cell infiltration of the connective tissue. Andreasen (1968) agreed with these criteria and regarded the presence of connective tissue inflammation as decisive. In a computer-aided analysis, Kramer et al. (1970*a*) listed the main criteria as hydropic and vacuolar degeneration of basal cells, epithelial atrophy, separation of epithelium from connective tissue, and inflammatory cell infiltration of the lamina propria. Lehner (1971) established that the distribution of inflammatory cell elements in the connective tissue characteristically differed between oral lichen and leukoplakia. McClatchey et al. (1975) described hyperkeratosis, acanthosis, hydropic degeneration of the stratum germinativum, an indistinct interface between epithelium and connective tissue, and a band-like inflammatory cell infiltration as the main histological features of lichen oris. Our histological observations generally agree with those of these authors.

In our experience, the occurrence of leukoplakia and lichen oris in the same site, either simultaneously or in sequence, is most possible. However, such co-existence at a common site in the 22 cases, observed in the present study, may have been as much due to chance as to a pathogenetic relationship and there is therefore no proof of the latter. Co-existence at different oral sites, as seen in five cases, implies neither a causal nor a pathogenetic relationship, and may also be a chance event.

Cancer development occurred in 5.9 (Bánóczy and L. Sugár 1972) and 0.4% (Kövesi and Bánóczy 1973*a*, *b*) of the total groups with leukoplakia and lichen oris, respectively, i.e. in 4.0% of the 846 cases combined in the two groups. Two cases of cancer development among 27 patients with coexistent lesions gives an incidence of 7.4%.

The small number of cases permits no definitive conclusions, but it seems that a combination of these two white lesions indicates a major risk of cancer.

INVESTIGATIONS OF WHITE SPONGE NAEVUS (LEUKOEDEMA EXFOLIATIVUM MUCOSAE ORIS)

The names "leukoedema exfoliativum mucosae oris" or "white sponge naevus" have been applied to a hereditary, dyskeratotic hyperplasia of the oral mucosa, a condition transmitted as an autosomal dominant trait (Scott 1966, Browne et al. 1969, Kamalamma et al. 1970). The lesions occur chiefly in oral epithelium, but occasionally the nasal, oesophageal, vaginal, anal or rectal mucosa also become involved (Ludy and Shirazy 1941, Bernstein and Lewin 1959, Cooke and Morgan 1959, Will 1966, Bánóczy 1968, Bánóczy and Sugár 1968, Haye and Whitehead 1968, Weiner 1969, L. Sugár and Bánóczy 1970, 1971, Ritzau 1971, Bánóczy et al. 1973,Hermann 1974).

This congenital dyskeratosis of the oral mucosa was first described by Cannon (1935), under the name "naevus spongiosus albus mucosae". Subsequently the condition was observed by several other authors, who variously termed it "leukokeratosis oris" (Ludy and Shirazy 1941), "white folded gingivostomatitis" (Orban and Wentz 1955, Everett and Noyes 1963), "pachydermia oralis" (Kinney and Derifield 1965), "white sponge naevus" (Bernstein and Lewin 1959, Smith 1962*b*, McCarthy and Shklar 1964), "soft leukoplakia" (Pashkov and Beljaeva 1966), or "naevus-like isolated hypertrophic keratosis of oral mucosa" (Will 1964). Case reports were also contributed by Cooke (1956), Darling and Fletcher (1958), Gaudy (1952), Zegarelli and Kutscher (1957), Zegarelli et al. (1959), Witkop and Gorlin (1961) and Scott (1966). Of the various names proposed, Cannon's original term "white sponge naevus" is still most widely used.

As far as we know, about 120 cases of white sponge naevus have so far been reported in the world literature. Our studies of the lesion have been described in several publications (Bánóczy and L. Sugár 1968*a*, L. Sugár and Bánóczy 1970*a*, 1971, Bánóczy et al. 1973).

Forty-five cases of white sponge naevus, seen in the Clinic of Maxillo-Facial Surgery and Dentistry, Dental Faculty of Semmelweis University Medical School, Budapest, over a period of 20 years, were examined by clinical, cyto-

Table 58

Age and sex distribution of white sponge naevus cases (leukoedema exfoliativum mucosae oris)

Age (years)	Men	Women	Total
<10	—	1	1
11–20	9	12	21
21–30	5	7	12
31–40	3	3	6
41–50	4	—	4
51–60	—	—	—
61–70	1	—	1
Totals	22	23	45

logical, histological and electron microscopic methods. The age and sex distribution of the patients is shown in Table 58.

The investigative methods were the same as in our studies of leukoplakia.

Specimens for electron microscopic examination were obtained from 13 patients, six men and seven women

Each specimen was fixed in 1% buffered OsO_4 (Rhodin 1954), dehydrated in ethanol, embedded in Epon, and cut in ultra-thin sections. These were counter-stained with 5% uranyl acetate (Watson 1958) and lead citrate (Karnovsky 1961), and examined in a Siemens Elmiscop I. The results have been published in detail (Frithiof and Bánóczy 1976*a*, *b*).

Clinical examinations

The condition had been present from a few weeks to 13 years as far as the patients knew. Twenty-eight patients were unaware of the lesion, which was either noticed by a dentist or found at screening for cancer. In no case could the history of the lesion traced back to infancy.

A familial incidence was observed in 12 cases: of these, the lesion was demonstrable in parents and children in seven cases, and among full sibs in four.

No relationship was demonstrated with any potential etiological factor. Eleven patients with a moderate smoking habit (8 to 10 cigarettes daily) showed no improvement of the lesion after temporary stopping the habit.

Twelve patients were habitual cheek-biters, and they had long held this responsible for the desquamation of their buccal epithelium. At clinical examination it was found that the lesion occurred not only in the cheeks, but also in other oral sites.

Clinical features: In the mobile mucous membrane large, slightly elevated, milk-white spots alternated with thickened epithelium desquamating in the form of scales, shreds, or thick patches. The shreds of epithelium could be removed by gentle rubbing; the underlying mucous membrane appeared intact, lacking any indication of haemorrhagic or inflammatory change. The gross appearance of the lesion was extraordinarily changeable: the patches of desquamating epithelium might nearly cover the entire mucosa one day and have practically disappeared by the next, only to reappear again within 2–3 days without any extraneous intervention. Adolescent patients usually showed more severe and extensive lesions than older ones. The lesions were limited to the loosely bound regions of oral mucosa: the main site was the cheek, in which 44 of the 45 patients had a lesion along the occlusal line. Next in frequency was the inner surface of the lips (19 cases), followed in the sequence by the tongue (15 cases), vestibule (7 cases) and floor of the mouth (3 cases). No lesions were found in the keratinizing epithelium of the gingiva and hard palate.

Several patients had a marked swelling of the fungiform papillae of the tongue (colour photos 14–16). Only a few patients also had lesion in other mucosae: two showed these at gynecological and four at laryngological examination. No patients had cutaneous symptoms, or any systemic change. Routine laboratory tests (RBC, WBC, ESR, barium test meal) revealed no abnormality.

Attempts to isolation fungi from the leukoedematous lesions were unsuccessful. Attempted treatments were prohibition of smoking, long-term general and local administration of large doses of vitamin A, hydrogen peroxide rinses, and topical Cortisol; none had any notable effect. Large doses of B vitamins did, however, provide temporary improvement.

Follow-up for 1–5 years in nine cases and for 5–10 years eight cases revealed neither regression, progression, nor malignant transformation. The benign nature of the lesion can also be deduced from the absence of malignant change in several generations of patients with a familial pattern of the disease.

Histological observations

Biopsies from 28 patients with white sponge naevus were examined histologically. The epithelium was thickened and extended broad processes into the connective tissue. The superficial layers of epithelium, 2–10 rows of cells, exhibited parakeratosis. All central epithelial layers had enlarged and oedematous cells. These cells had a clear cytoplasm, without lipid inclusions, and a shrunken nucleus, placed either centrally or peripherally, which disappeared

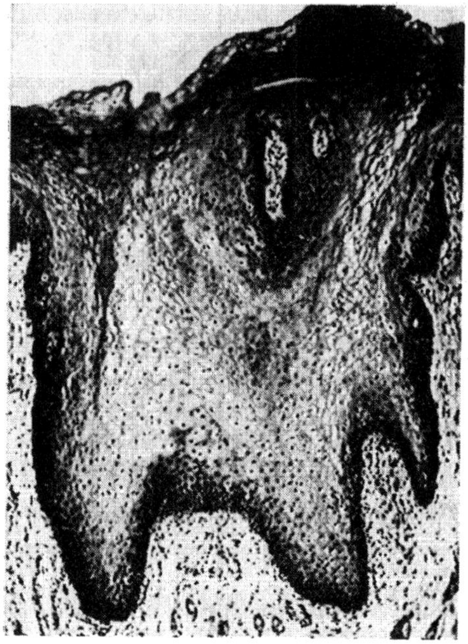

Fig. 111. Microscopic appearance of white sponge naevus. Note thickening of the parakeratotic layers. The spinous cells are vacuolated and there are indications of spongiosis and intercellular separation. There is no inflammatory cell reaction in the connective tissue. H. & E., ×120

altogether in the most advanced stages of oedema. The ballon-like hydropic degeneration of epithelium at first appeared to involve only single cells or groups of cells, but later many cell boundaries became indefinite and microscopic intra-epithelial spaces were formed. The basal layer of epithelium was never involved in hydropic change. The epithelial–connective tissue interface remained sharply demarcated. No epithelial layer showed any indication of pre-malignant or malignant change. The subepithelial connective tissue was either slightly inflamed or uninflamed (Fig. 111).

Cytological observations

In 23 cases cytological smears were taken and examined by the method of Papanicolaou and Traut (1943). Witkop and Gorlin (1961) described a relative increase in keratinized cells and the "cell within cell" phenomenon as the main cytological characteristics of white sponge naevus. The term "cell within cell" refers to the presence of eosinophilic or orangeophilic cytoplasmic aggregations pushing the nucleus to one side. Such cells should be acidophilic, dyskeratotic forms. We did not see them in our cytological smears, but a quantitative increase of keratinized cells was obvious. Alterations in the quantitative distribution of epithelial cells in relation to normal oral mucosa are shown in Table 59.

Table 59

Proportions of keratinized cells from different oral sites in patients with white sponge naevus

Site		No. of cases	Normal and leukoedematous oral mucosa	
Cheek	blue	23	83.5	35
	red		11.7	25
	yellow		4.8	40
Dorsum of tongue	blue	8	52.7	35.5
	red		32.2	26.5
	yellow		13.1	43
Labial inner surface	blue	10	67	29
	red		27	31
	yellow		6	40

As can be seen, the number of keratinized cells was increased in smears taken from loosely bound sites, while the cell distribution was normal in smears from regions lined by tightly bound, keratinizing epithelium.

Most smears took on a characteristic pale stain. The keratinized cells did not assume the vivid orange shade seen in normal smears or in other keratinizing lesions. Nearly all keratinized cells had pyknotic nuclei (colour photo 17). Keratohyaline granules were seen within non-keratinized cells in only two cases; these were indicative of parakeratosis. All smears contained many bacteria and leukocytes. In 12 smears there was a marked paucity of cells.

Electron microscopic observations

The basement membrane region. The epithelial–connective tissue interface was generally smooth, with epithelial ridges arising from a broad base. Epithelium was separated from connective tissue by a lamina lucida, and by a continuous basement membrane of normal thickness and structure. Stratification of the basement membrane in some areas was seen in eight cases (Fig. 112). The connective tissue contained collagen fibres and fibroblasts, but very few inflammatory cells. Mast cells were found in three cases. (Frithiof and Bánóczy 1976*a*).*

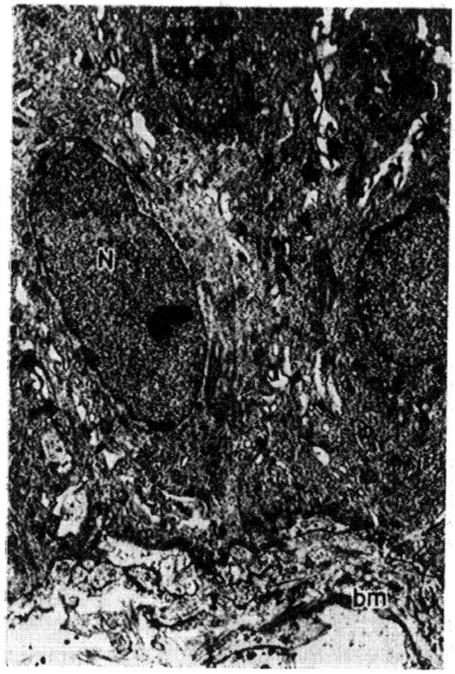

Fig. 112. White sponge naevus: Lower part of the basal and spinous layers. Note multi-layered basement membrane. The intercellular space is of normal width. The number of tonofilaments is increased, the nuclear membrane is smooth. bm = basement membrane, N = nucleus. ×6,000

Stratum basale. The basal cells were cylindrical and their laminar surface adjoining the basement membrane was fairly smooth. Many hemidesmosomes could be seen.

The cell surface facing the narrow intercellular spaces was irregular, with thin cytoplasmic processes. Desmosomes furnishing the intercellular junctions were supported by broad processess containing tonofilaments. The distribution of cytoplasmic tonofilaments, ribosomes and mitochondria was characteristic of moderately keratinized epithelium. The tonofilaments were usually aggregated into boundles which were directly associated with desmosomes.

The nuclei were round or oval, with a generally smooth but occasionally irregular surface. The nuclear chromatin was evenly distributed and the nucleoli were conspicuous.

In some specimens there were irregular basal cells with a markedly vacuolated cytoplasm and a folded nuclear membrane (Fig. **113**). Such cells contained an increased number of mitochondria.

Stratum spinosum. The cells and nuclei of the stratum spinosum equally showed gradual increase in size. Cells of the lower row(s) contained

Fig. 113. White sponge naevus: Irregular, abundantly vacuolated basal cells. The nuclear membrane is irregular. The basement membrane shows no stratification. bm = basement membrane, N = nucleus, v = vacuole. ×6,000

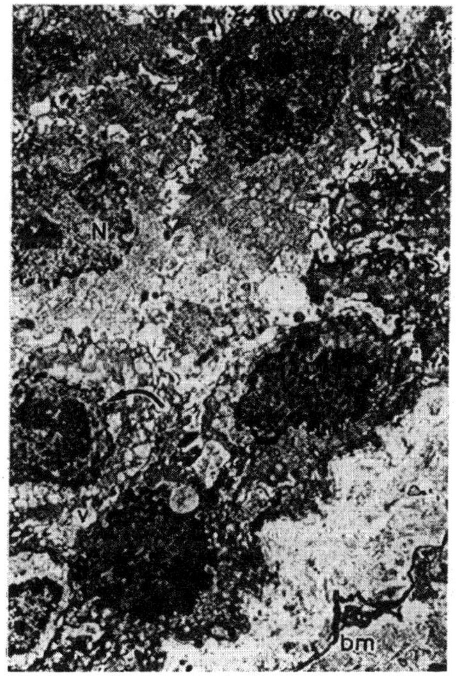

dispersed tonofilaments, which gave them a homogeneous appearance (Fig. 114). In the central and superficial rows tonofilaments were aggregated in one part of the cell, where there were few ribosomes, these organelles were aggregated in another part, where many mitochondria were also present. Intracellular glycogen granules occurred in a third part, sharply demarcated from the other organelles (Fig. 115). Intracellular areas without organelles were also seen in most preparations. A total of 12 specimens showed these changes in the stratum spinosum.

The concentration of tonofilaments was considerably greater than in normal buccal mucosa (see Fig. 115). Tonofilaments were aggregated into bundles chiefly in basal cells, and this pattern largely disappeared in the lower rows of the stratum spinosum, which consequently did not contain tonofibrils, not even near to desmosomes.

Marked segregation of organelles, and a homogeneous distribution of tonofilaments were the most typical features of cells in the stratum spinosum.

Four specimens showed an unusual, and previously unobserved pattern of tonofilament bundles. At magnifications of less than ×10,000 these aggregations were reminiscent of the roundish shape of keratohyaline gran-

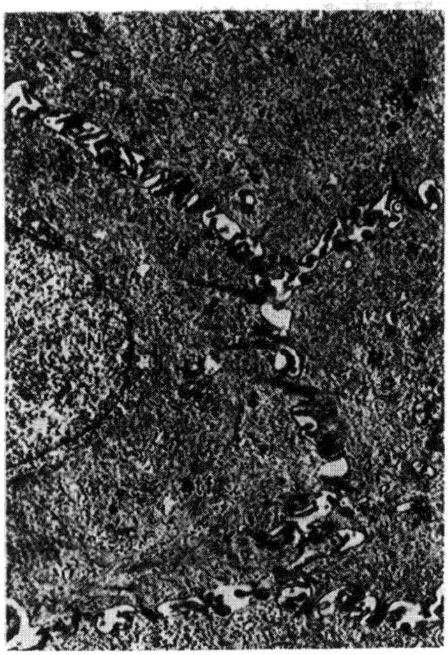

Fig. 114. White sponge naevus: Lower part of the stratum spinosum. The cells are enlarged with a structurally homogeneous cytoplasm. There are many tonofilaments and desmosomes. tf = tonofilament, d = desmosome, N = nucleus. ×9,000

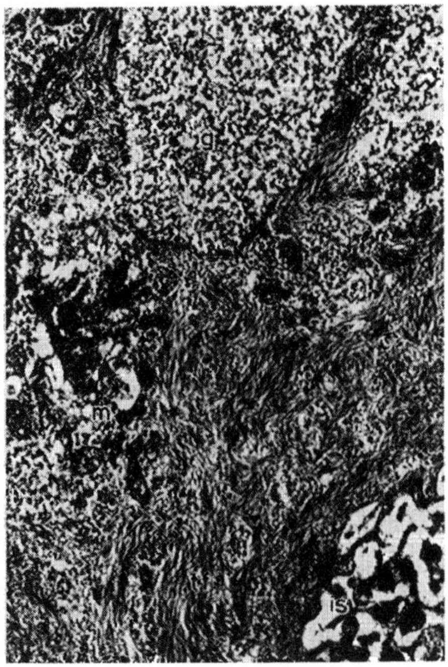

Fig. 115. White sponge naevus: Central part of the stratum spinosum. Note segregation of the organelles into different intracellular compartments. Glycogen is accumulated in the upper part of the cell, the ribosomes and mitochondria are in another part, away from the tonofilaments. Note intercellular space with many desmosomes at bottom right. g = glycogen, tf = tonofilament, m = mitochondrion, is = intercellular space. ×18,000

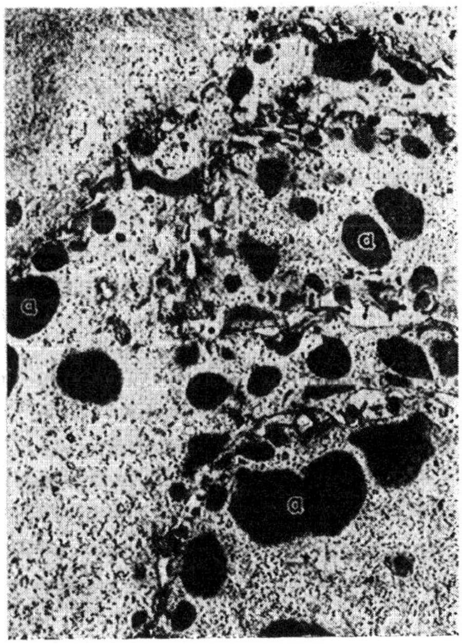

Fig. 116. White sponge naevus: Upper part of the stratum spinosum. Aggregation of tonofilaments forms many round, electron-dense bodies. Some aggregations are linked with the desmosomes by tonofilaments. a = electron-dense aggregation. ×9,000

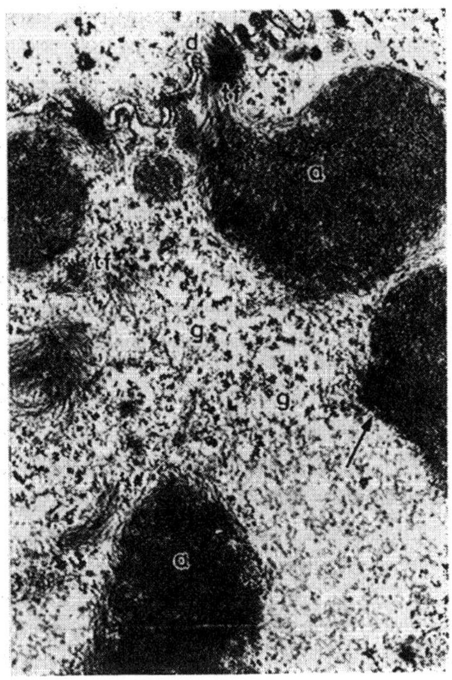

Fig. 117. White sponge naevus: Electron micrograph of the electron-dense aggregation. Its components can be easily identified as tonofilaments at this level of magnification. d = desmosome, tf = tonofilament, a = aggregation, g = glycogen. ×30,000

ules (Fig. 116), but were less electron dense than them, and also of different structure. They were located near to the cell boundary and were frequently attached to desmosomes by tonofilaments. Their filamentous margins could be recognized at low magnification (Fig. 116), and at a higher resolution the longitudinal and transverse cross-sections of the tonofilaments also became visible (Fig. 117).

Unlike normal buccal mucosa, white sponge naevus contained many Odland bodies (Odland 1960), with a distinct lamellar structure (Figs 118 and 119). However, lamellar bodies were only occasionally present in the intercellular spaces. Small keratohyaline granules occurred in only two specimens.

Some cells located in the upper part of the stratum spinosum showed signs of cytoplasmic degeneration and contained only a few peripheral aggregations of filaments (Fig. 120). Their nuclear structure had lost definition, although the nuclear membrane was generally preserved. Complete cell destruction was, however, observed in only one specimen.

Stratum superficiale. The thickness of the flat-cell layer was variable. The degree of keratinization did not always follow a sequential pattern. This groups of parakeratotic cells were often present in the lower rows, while keratinization was less pronounced in the upper layers.

The superficial cells were either parakeratotic or non-keratinized. There was no sign of orthokeratosis. In some sections the surface was covered by structureless, flat cells.

Accumulation of bacteria on the epithelial surface was obvious in all specimens except two (Fig. 121). Bacteria had also invaded the intercellular spaces beneath the superficial rows and some had even penetrated intracellularly.

The age and sex distribution of our patients with white sponge naevus was similar to that observed by other. The lesion is usually detected during childhood or puberty. Our 63-year-old patient was an exception, as only four other cases have been reported in the world literature in that age group (Cannon 1935, Bernstein and Lewin 1959, Scott 1966, Ritzau 1971). A familial incidence was demonstrated in 25% of our cases, but it may have been greater as many patients were unaware of their lesions and their blood relatives were not available for study.

The clinical appearance of the lesions was described in many publications. The change was more pronounced in younger than in older patients. Cooke (1956), Scott (1966), and Browne et al. (1969) believed that the white sponge naevus tends to progress up to a certain age and then becomes static. As to the site of the lesion, it occurred chiefly in the buccal, lingual and labial mucosa and never in regions without a submucosa, although lesions on the gingiva and hard palate have been reported in the literature (Cannon 1935,

Fig. 118. White sponge naevus: Upper part of the stratum spinosum. There is no tonofibril formation: some tonofilaments are scattered in the cytoplasm, others form peripheral aggregations. Note the Odland bodies, 0.1 to 0.2 μ in diameter, in marginal parts of the cells. a = aggregation, o = Odland bodies. ×6,000

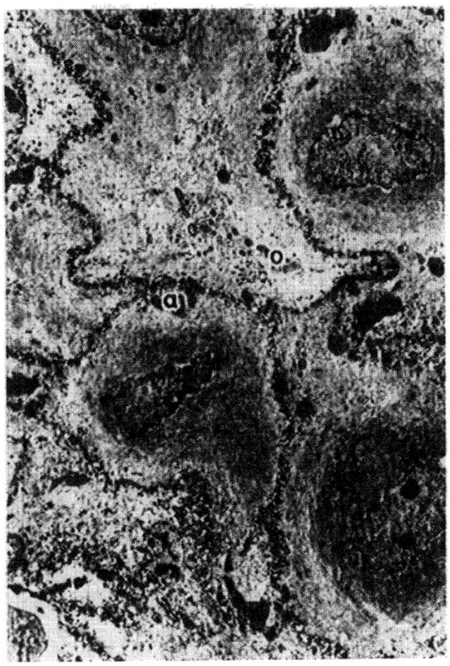

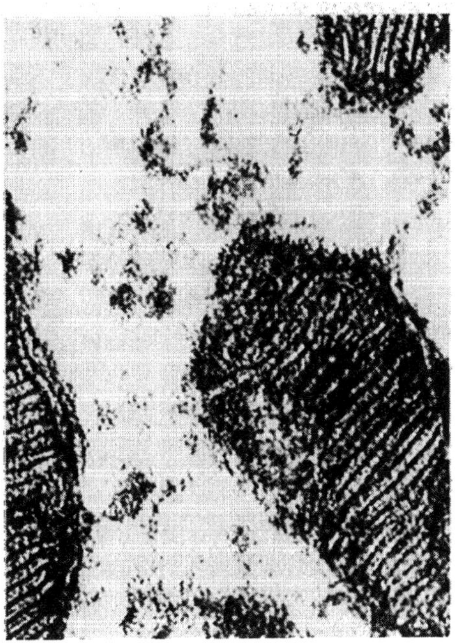

Fig. 119. White sponge naevus: Odland bodies. ×240,000

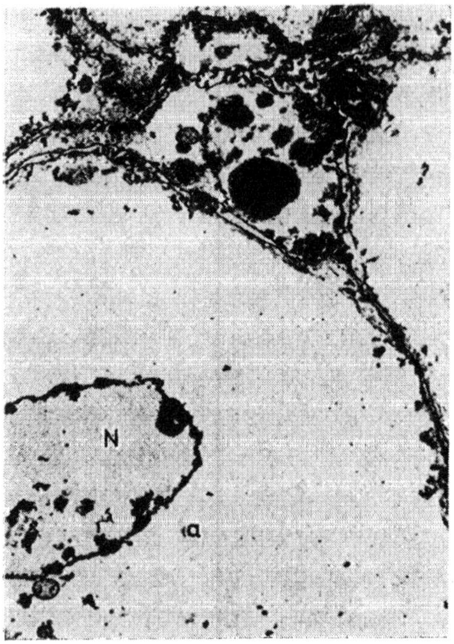

Fig. 120. White sponge naevus: Disintegrating spinous cell. There are a few electron-dense aggregations of tonofilaments at the cell periphery. N = nucleus, a = aggregation. ×6,000

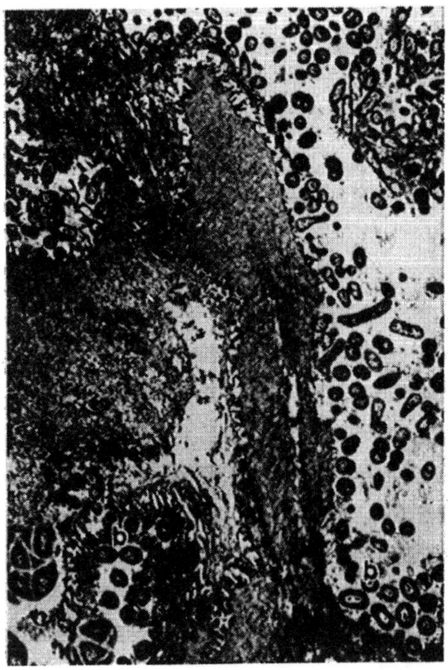

Fig. 121. White sponge naevus: Epithelial surface. Plaque-like depositions of bacteria are also present in the intercellular spaces between superficial cells. b = bacterium. ×6,000

Ludy and Shirazy 1941, Bernstein and Lewin 1959, Scott 1966, Weiner 1969 and Ritzau 1971).

The extremely thick parakeratotic layers seen in the histological sections may be the result of retarded desquamation due to deficient or delayed detachment of desmosomes. Keratohyaline granules were either absent or present in very small numbers. Complete keratinization with orthokeratosis was not seen. The deficient, incomplete keratinization may have been due to marked spongiosis of the stratum spinosum.

Our cytological observation of a quantitative increase of keratinized cells corresponds with that of Witkop and Gorlin (1961), but we failed to detect the eosinophilic cytoplasmic condensations described by them. The paucity of cells in the cytological smears can be attributed to reduced desquamation.

The differentiation of white sponge naevus from leukoplakia has presented a major diagnostic problem. The two conditions are frequently confused; of our 45 patients with white sponge naevus 28 had originally been referred to our clinical department with a diagnosis of oral leukoplakia. Leukoplakia usually occurs at a more advanced age than the naevus, the lesion is more sharply demarcated, and some irritating factor is as a rule demonstrable. Two patients were referred to us with a diagnosis of lichen oris; this lesion is not desquamative and displays the characteristic striae of Wickham. Candidiasis may also give to a "white lesion" in the mouth; it is also identified by a lack of desquamation, and, above all, by positive isolation of the fungus. The rare condition termed "leukoedema" by Sandstead and Lowe (1953) may also be mistaken for white sponge naevus on clinical inspection, but can be differentiated from it with certainty by histological examination.

Since ultrastructural studies of white sponge naevus have been done only by Whitten (1970) in five cases, it seemed worth-while to analyze in a greater detail our electron microscopic observations of 13 subjects.

The reason for the stratification of basement membrane, which was observed in several cases, remains obscure. Frithiof (1969) found a similar change, associated with inflammatory infiltration of adjacent connective tissue epithelial hyperplasia and in so-called "benign" forms of leukoplakia. in However, there is little if any inflammation of the subepithelial connective tissue in white sponge naevus. Multiplication of the basement membrane is probably indicative of increased epithelial activity in this condition.

The presence of two structurally different types of basal cells may signify a cyclic pattern of epithelial activity. The concentration of tonofilaments in basal cells usually exceeded that present in normal buccal or vestibular epithelium, but was still less than that found in epithelium of the gingiva and hard palate. The bundle-like aggregations of tonofilaments are seen as an intermediate or transitional stage between keratinized and non-keratinized oral epithelium.

Unlike normal keratinizing epithelium, the stratum spinosum of the naevus had dispersed tonofilaments, which imparted to it the particular "homogeneous" appearance which was also noticed by Whitten (1970). Brody (1960) demonstrated tonofibrils in normal spinous cells, which may be entirely absent in leukoedema.

Other characteristic features of the stratum spinosum of white sponge naevus, such as the segregation of intracellular filaments, ribosomes and glycogen in different compartments, and the clumping of tonofilaments found in four cases also indicate a severe cellular dysfunction. The clumping is not confined to white sponge naevus, as it has also been observed (Ishibashi and Klingmüller 1968) in three cases of erythrodermia ichthyosiformis congenita bullosa Brocq (EICB), where it was interpreted as a sequel to cytochemical dysfunction. It should be noted, however, that neither dispersion of filaments nor segregation of organelles was found in EICB.

The normal human non-keratinizing buccal and vestibular epithelium (Frithiof and Wersäll 1965, Gemell and Chapman 1971, El-Labban and Kramer 1974*a*, *b*) does not usually contain Odland bodies either in intra- or intercellular sites. Such bodies are a feature of keratinizing cells (Frithiof 1970). Wolff and Holubar (1968), as well as Luzardo-Baptista and Garcia-Tamayo (1971*c*) associated alkaline phosphatase activity with the Odland bodies and concluded that extracellular phosphatase promotes the desquamation of epithelial cells.

The presence of many Odland bodies in the parakeratotic buccal mucosa of patients with leukoedema suggests that the granules are related to the process of keratinization. The fact that only a few Odland bodies enter the intercellular space in leukoedema indicates a different pattern from normal keratinization.

If the conclusion reached by Luzardo-Baptista and Garcia-Tamayo (1971*c*) is correct, absence of the lamellar substance from the intercellular space would explain the marked accumulation of superficial cells in white sponge naevus. Desmosomes, which almost certainly account for the maintenance of intercellular junctions, also are more numerous in the lesion than in normal non-keratinizing epithelium (Frithiof 1972).

The formation of a bacterial "plaque" on the epithelial surface could well be the result of retarded desquamation. When the rate of desquamation is normal, colonization of the epithelial surface does not usually take place.

MORSICATIO BUCCARUM ET LABIORUM: A CLINICOPATHOLOGICAL EXAMINATION

During the last 15 years several authors have separated the white lesion which is caused by habitual cheek-biting (morsicatio buccarum) from other lesions of the oral mucosa because its etiology is known and it has well-defined clinical and histological features (Schuermann 1958, Kocsárd et al. 1962, Obermayer 1964, Vakilzadek 1967). Hjorting-Hansen and Holst (1970) as well as Sewerin (1971) studied the condition in 17 and 42 patients, respectively. We described in a previous publication (Sonkodi and Bánóczy 1974) the clinical and histological characteristics and the treatment of 32 patients with the condition, 19 of whom had been seen in the Maxillo-Facial Surgery and Dentistry Departments of the University Medical School of Szeged and 13 in the same clinics in Budapest. In this chapter studies of 18 cases of cheek-biting are described, selected from among the patients seen in the Oral Disease Department of the Clinic of Maxillo-Facial Surgery and Dentistry, Semmelweis University Medical School, Budapest, over a 6-year period from 1968 to 1974.

The age and sex distribution of the patients is shown in Table 60.

There were ten men and eight women and two-thirds of these patients were in the age range 10 to 29 years.

Three *forms* of the lesion could be distinguished by their gross appearance. The most frequent change was the presence of scraps of white-greyish epithelium, not removed by rubbing, in the bitten area (Fig. 122). Less often there was a prominent ridge of whitish mucosa along the occlusal line (Fig. 123), or occasionally erosions or even ulcerations were present (Fig. 124) at the bitten site.

Table 60

Age and sex distribution of morsicatio buccarum et labiorum (cheek-biting)

Age (years)	Men	Women	Totals
10–19	1	3	4
20–29	5	3	8
30–39	—	—	—
40–49	3	—	3
50–59	1	1	2
>60	—	1	1
Totals	10	8	18

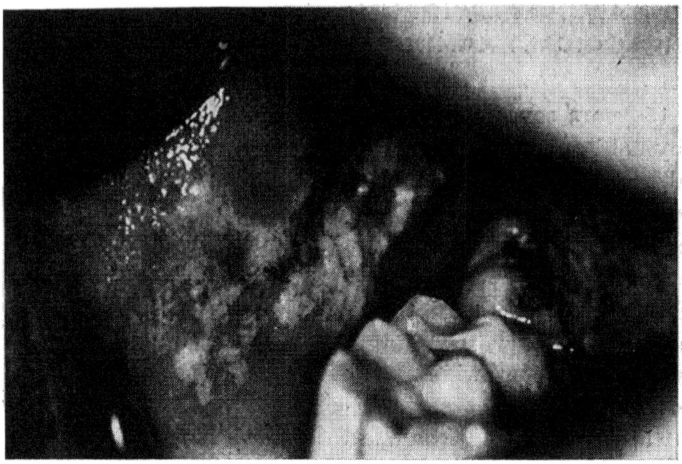

Fig. 122. Lesion of morsicatio buccarum (cheek-biting) in a 14-year-old girl. White-greyish shreds of epithelial tissue, not removable by rubbing, can be seen on the buccal mucosa

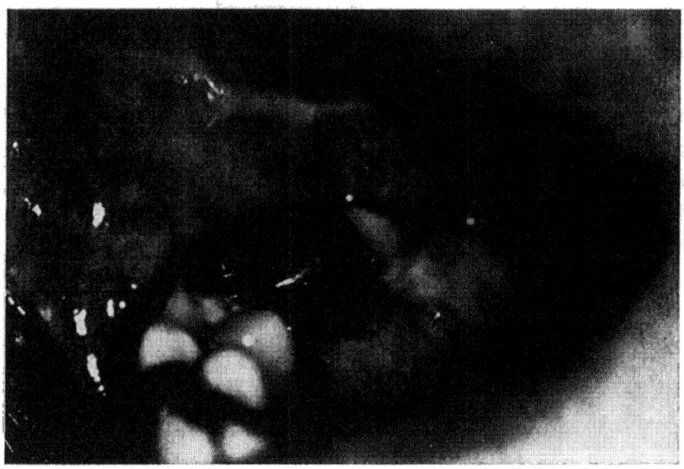

Fig. 123. Lesion of morsicatio buccarum (cheek-biting) lesion in a 40-year-old male patient. Note the ridge in the buccal mucosa along the occlusal line

The lesion(s) were usually found on the buccal and labial mucosa, less often at the commissures, as a rule, bilaterally.

As to the *etiology* of the lesion, eight of the 18 patients were aware of habitual biting of the cheek or lip. They knew that their habit had been present

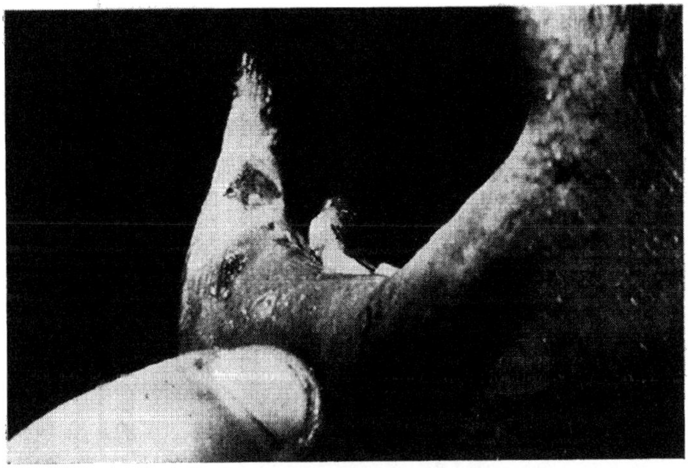

Fig. 124. Lesion of morsicatio labiorum (lip.biting) in a 23-year-old neurotic male patient. Continuous biting gave rise to ulcerations in the commissures, and on the inner surface of the lower lip

from 1–5 years. As to the reason for adopting this habit, most patients attributed it to some form of psychological conflict. A neurotic 23-year-old male, referred to our Department from the Neurology and Psychiatry Clinic, reported that several members of his family were also psychologically disturbed, and that his cheek-biting habit was motivated by attempts to control his nervous impulses (see Fig. 124).

In one case cheek-biting lesion was associated with lichen oris and in three cases with leukoedema exfoliativum mucosae oris. Four patients only had a moderate smoking habit, and fungal infection and a high electric potential difference were each found in a single case.

Histological appearance. The epithelium was hyperplastic and coated by a thin layer of bacteria. Hyperparakeratosis was present without a distinct stratum granulosum. Hyperplasia of the stratum spinosum gave rise to acanthosis, accompanied by spongiosis and hydropic degeneration, which also occurred in a less pronounced form in the basal layer. There was no sign of pre-malignant change, and the basement membrane was intact. The connective tissue showed a very mild, predominantly lymphocytic, inflammatory cell infiltration (Fig. 125).

The *treatment* of morsicatio buccarum et labiorum centered chiefly on psychotherapy. Sharp-edged teeth smoothed, and/or acrylic splints were fitted. Three patients were cured of the habit, five showed improvement, but the remaining ten either did not return for treatment, or disregarded the proposed therapy.

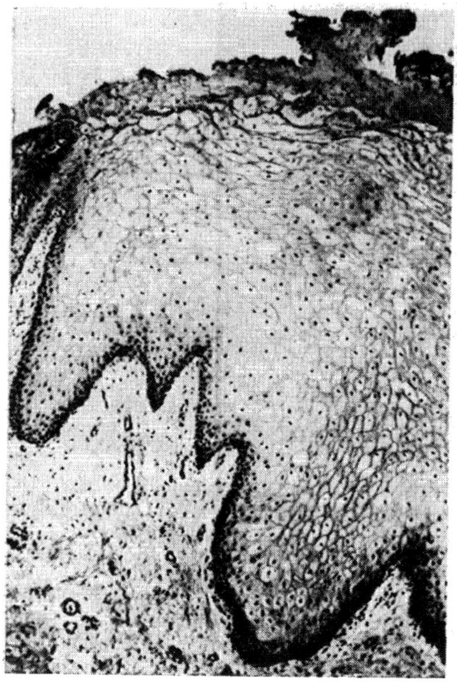

Fig. 125. Microscopic appearance of a lesion caused by cheek-biting. The epithelium is thick and acanthotic. The superficial layer is hyperparakeratotic, the stratum spinosum cells show a hydropic degeneration. The subepithelial connective tissue shows a very slight inflammatory cell reaction. H. & E., ×125

The period of observation ranged from 1 to 6 years; no malignant transformation occurred during that time.

The prevalence of cheek-biting was found to be 1.05% among textile mill workers (Sonkodi and Bánóczy 1974), 0.48% among selected dental patients (Sewerin 1971), and 4.7% in a random population group in Sweden (Axell 1975).

The age-group distribution of our patients corresponded with that observed by Hjorting-Hansen and Holst (1970) and by Sewerin (1971). The prevalence of the condition in young subjects is presumably related to the presence of an intact dentition; the incidence of cheek-biting decreases with age, as the dentition is so often depleted by caries and periodontal disease. As to the site of the lesion, we agree with Sewerin (1971) that the buccal mucosa is the most commonly affected site.

Investigations have usually shown the etiological significance of psychological instability and Kocsárd et al. (1962), Obermayer (1964), Schuermann (1958) and Sewerin (1971) found that most patients could be classified as intellectuals. This observation can be applied to the group that we studied, but in a previous study (Sonkodi and Bánóczy 1974) 19 patients were industrial workers which indicates that psychological change elicited by stress is not confined to intellectuals.

Obermayer (1964) described in a case report the superimposition of morsicatio buccarum et labiorum on white sponge naevus. Among the 19 cases seen by us, cheek-biting was associated with lichen oris in one case, and white sponge naevus in three cases. Nervous patients are liable to bite pathologically altered parts of their oral mucous membrane. Among our 45 patients with white sponge naevus 13 (28.8%) admitted to such a habit (Bánóczy et al. 1973) but, as also shown by Sewerin (1971), most cheek-biting patients originally had intact oral mucosa.

Among the patients referred to our Department from other medical institutions five had been diagnosed as having oral leukoplakia, and one oral lichen. The differential diagnosis of cheek-biting includes candidiasis and white sponge naevus. Grossly the lesion is reminiscent of oral candidiasis, but parts of the lesion cannot be removed by scraping and the fungus cannot be demonstrated microscopically. Differentiation from oral leukoplakia depends on the presence of the clear-cut etiological factor (of cheek-biting), from lichen by the absence of typical clinical signs such as Wickham's striae and a papular distribution and by histological differences, and from white sponge naevus by absence of a familial incidence.

Cheek-biting lesions showed no tendency to malignant transformation. Schuermann et al. (1966) have classified morsicatio buccarum et labiorum as a symptomatic leukoplakia, and a precancerous condition following upon traumatic irritation. Most other authors, including ourselves, agree that it is essentially benign.

CHAPTER VIII

THE THERAPY OF ORAL LEUKOPLAKIA

A review of various approaches to therapy and their results is an integral part of any clinical study. The therapeutic aspect is especially important in those conditions in which treatment of a basic disorder prevents a more serious outcome, such as malignant change in oral leukoplakia.

It therefore seems appropriate to survey the literature on the therapy of leukoplakia, together with present knowledge and our own experience of those treatments to which the condition is most responsive. Some important aspects of our therapeutic approach have already been described (Bánóczy 1964, 1965*a*, *b*, L. Sugár and Bánóczy 1957, 1959, 1969, Bánóczy and L. Sugár 1968*b*, Bánóczy 1977).

Leukoplakia may be treated (*i*) conservatively, (*ii*) by surgical excision, (*iii*) by irradiation, or by a combination of these methods.

Investigators engaged in the study of oral leukoplakia disagree on many points, but they generally agree that the success of any treatment depends upon the elimination of any predisposing factors. It is therefore imperative to prohibit smoking, to remove bad teeth, and to exchange faulty metal restorations and/or metal bridges responsible for electric potential differences before any other treatment. Not infrequently elimination of irritating factor(s) will effect complete healing. After Balogh (1956), such lesions are called reversible. In gross appearance reversible lesions generally are either wrinkled, lustreless patches with a slight and diffuse keratinization, or a mosaic-like plaque. Conservative or surgical treatment is indicated if (*i*) elimination of the etiological factors is not followed by healing within 2–3 weeks, i.e. the lesion is irreversible, or (*ii*) if there is no demonstrable etiological factor, or (*iii*) if the lesion progresses to papillary proliferation or ulceration (verrucous or erosive leukoplakia).

As a *conservative treatment,* administration of vitamin A has been preferred because of the known protective effect of the vitamin on epithelium. Deficiency of vitamin A leads to keratinization in normally non-keratinizing regions of the oral mucosa and also to metaplasia of secretory columnar epithelium to keratinizing squamous epithelium (Hyams and Bloom 1947). The daily vitamin A requirement of man is 4,000 IU, but the treatment of hyperkeratosis requires considerably higher doses, administered on a continuous schedule. Mulay and Urbach (1958) were the first to use vitamin A for the topical therapy of oral leukoplakia. Later, Smith (1962*a*) gave 75,000–300,000 IU daily by mouth for periods of 3–18 months. 72% of slightly hyperkeratotic lesions and only 25% of massively keratotic and ulcerative forms improved under the influence of vitamin A, and the histologically dyskeratotic and pre-malignant lesions were unresponsive. Signs of hypervitaminosis were not observed. Silverman et al. (1963*a*, *b*) reported that short-term, large-dose treatment with vitamin A (300,000–900,000 IU daily) leads to the improvement of hyperkeratosis, but its withdrawal was followed by relapse. Kovács (1962*a*) obtained good therapeutic results with long-term oral or parenteral doses of 100,000 IU vitamin A daily, in combination with vitamin E, to inhibit its metabolic degradation. During recent years Swiss and mostly German clinicians have experimented with a large-dose vitamin A therapy. Spiessl and Metz (1957) observed improvement of oral leukoplakia on treatment with vitamin A at a daily dose of 100,000–150,000 IU. Short-term treatment with subtoxic doses of vitamin A-palmitate (Esser 1972), with aromatic retinoids (Ehrl 1980) or all-trans-β-A-vitamin acid plus 13-cis-β-A-vitamin acid (Koch and Schettler 1973) was followed by healing or improvement in some cases.

Untoward side-effects and the possibility of relapse upon withdrawal have, however, prevented the wide application of subtoxic vitamin A therapy for the time being. Recently Brunner (1975) reported recurrence of oral leukoplakia after short-term cure with subtoxic vitamin A dosis.

In the 'sixties animal experiments (Levij and Polliack 1968, Polliack and Levij 1969) and clinical studies (Odens 1961) supported the view that, through enhancement of membrane permeability, vitamin A might promote the intracellular penetration of carcinogens. Cell culture studies (Lucy and Dingle 1964, Dingle and Lucy 1965, Weissman 1965, Basset and Pacher 1965, Brandes and Anton 1966, Dingle et al. 1966, Bánóczy and Török 1972) have shown that, through enhancement of the membrane permeability of lysosomes, released lysosomal enzymes may also promote both the intracellular penetration of carcinogens and oncogenesis. In view of these observations, great caution has been recently exercised in planning vitamin A therapy of oral leukoplakia, particularly by the oral and parenteral routes.

Successful topical treatment of oral leukoplakia has been reported to occur after painting the lesions with podophyllin solution (Kovács 1962*a*). Podophyllin seems to act through its ability to inhibit mitosis.

The association of candidiasis with oral leukoplakia has been known since the related investigations of Jepsen and Winther (1965) and Balogh and Lelkes (1965). Since then candidiasis has been acknowledged as one of the etiological factors in oral leukoplakia. According to Cawson (1966), candidiasis gives rise to parakeratosis, and on deeper penetration to dyskeratosis, which may become irreversible after a certain time. Hahn and Lange (1967) and Pindborg et al. (1968) have agreed that the "speckled" type of leukoplakia is frequently associated with a candidiasis, and that the treatment of such cases with Nystatin may result in clinical improvement.

In the Clinic of Maxillo-Facial Surgery and Dentistry, Dental Faculty of Semmelweis University Medical School, Budapest, oral leukoplakia is treated by conservative methods if (*i*) elimination of etiological factors fails to bring about a remission of an initially mild lesion, or if (*ii*) a reduction in size of the changed area is deemed necessary before the surgical excision of, for example, extensive verrucous lesions.

As to the use of vitamin A therapy, we have been obliged to change our mind in the course of our long-term studies. While formerly we preferred large oral doses (3×15 drops of oily emulsion, 9–12 dragées, or 2×1 capsules, each 50,000 IU) for a period of 2–3 months, recently we have used vitamin A chiefly by local application, either in combination or alternately with ointments which enhance epithelization.

If there is bacteriological evidence of candidiasis, elimination of predisposing factors, such as curtailing the use of a prosthesis is combined with intensive Nystatin therapy (2×1 tablets, i.e. $2 \times 500{,}000$ IU daily), plus painting with a solution of 20% borax-glycerol or 1% gentian violet, and/or mouth rinses with a $1 >$ chlorogen solution. The antimycotic preparations Canesten and Pimafucin have also been effective. A cure by vaccination may be attempted in the case of infection by a resistant strain.

Complementary treatment with vitamins of the B complex is particularly helpful in the case of commissural and lingual lesions. Treatment with vitamin B_{12} is imperative if the condition is associated with anaemia. The use of Panthenol lingual tablets or Panthenol oral spray has been also effective against complaints such as glossitis and glossodynia.

The question may be justly put as to which cases require conservative treatment and which necessitate surgical intervention.

It is generally agreed that *surgical intervention* should be contemplated only if conservative therapy fails, but no-one except Hollander and co-workers (1933) have specified the criteria of failure. These authors recommended electro-coagulation of the lesion if 14 days of conservative treatment has no effect. Smith (1962*a*) displayed more patience, stating that vitamin A therapy takes 4–6 months to have the desired effect. Vándor (1969) held the view that long observation and constant conservative therapy of leukoplakia and delayed surgical intervention often cause progress of the lesion until the stage of malignant transformation.

If conservative treatment fails, leukoplakia may (*i*) either be removed radically by surgical excision, or (*ii*) sequential biopsies may be taken if there is no evidence of malignant change.

Radical surgery has been advocated chiefly by Anglo-Saxon authors (Bradley 1956, Kwapis and Gibson 1956, Brown 1962), who have preferred total excision to biopsy regardless of the clinical type, in order to prevent malignant transformation.

Welsh (1955) suggested that biopsy is necessary if an originally diffuse leukoplakia transforms to the verrucous type or to what he calls "leukokeratosis". Roumanian authors (Engels et al. 1958) advocated the histological monitoring of leukokeratosis and of recurrent lesions. German authors have selected the surgical method by clinical type. Mathis (1964) and Rosenthal (1962) preferred the total surgical excision of verrucous leukoplakia, and Rosenthal (1962) warned against tampering with biopsies instead of total excision once a fissure or a growth was present. Fasske et al. (1959*c*) preferred the total excision of all lesions classified by them as grade IV (35% prevalence of malignant transformation). With lesions classified as "diffuse" by clinical appearance, elimination of irritating factor(s) and continuous observation may be sufficient, but histological examination should be performed in suspicious cases. Rosenthal (1962) and Boyle (1954) referred the taking of biopsies to a competent surgical specialist who may also take charge of the radical excision, should histological findings disclose indications of malignancy. Authors generally agree that observation should be continued after radical surgery, for intervention eliminates the lesion, but not the individual disposition to leukoplakia. The existence of such a predisposition was supported by the observation of Fasske et al (1959*a*, *b*) that in a substantial number of the cases, leukoplakia arises without any obvious cause. Meyer and Shklar (1960), Sharp et al. (1961) and Sharp (1956) concluded from studies on large groups of patients that since those with oral carcinoma had other abnormal areas of oral mucous membrane with both atrophic and leukoplakic changes, the unicentric theory of carcinogenesis should be superceded by one that allows for multicentric origin within extensively altered abnormal epithelium. Similar opinions have been expressed by Moertel and Foss (1958), Moertel et al. (1961), Bodart (1968), Allmen (1978), and Burkhardt and Seifert (1977). The possibility of a leukoplakic disposition was also considered by Winiker-Blanck (1961), who recommended prolonged postoperative supervision on the grounds that among 47 patients subjected to radical surgery for leukoplakia, seven showed recurrence of the lesion within 5 years.

Certain authors (Knychalska-Karwan 1965*b*, Rehrmann and Pape 1966, Schwenzer 1968, Matras 1969, Symeonidis 1969, Rennefarth and Kunze 1969, Tempel 1972, Gombos et al. 1974, Allmen 1978) have unconditionally advocated the surgical removal of all types of leukoplakia.

The new technique of cryosurgery has recently been employed for intraoral operations (Poswillo 1971). The full range of indications for its use have yet to be established (Leopard and Poswillo 1974), but it seems suitable for the radical removal of previously untreated precancerous oral lesions (Sonkodi and Keszthelyi 1975). The promising results obtained in Hungary with the cryotherapy of oral leukoplakias have been described in detail by Sonkodi (1976).

In the Clinic of Maxillo-Facial Surgery and Dentistry, Dental Faculty of Semmelweis University Medical School, Budapest, surgery has generally been used for the removal of verrucous, erosive or ulcerated leukoplakias of small size. Accordingly, small, circumscribed leukoplakias of the cheek and tongue are excised, while those located on the hard palate or alveolar ridge are treated by electrocoagulation.

For large leukoplakias, whose excision would involve unnecessary destruction of tissue, usually an explorative biopsy is first taken. If histological examination reveals indications of malignancy, either radical surgery or radiation therapy is employed. If there is no histological evidence of malignancy, but the lesion is of the verrucous or erosive type, local treatment with vitamin A is used to achieve a reduction in size, after which the lesion must be excised eventually in stages at several operations.

The opponents of surgical treatment believe that since the development of leukoplakia depends greatly on individual predisposition and on extensive alteration of the oral epithelium, the surgical excision of the lesion cannot prevent its recurrence. We partly agree with this view, since idiopathic forms of leukoplakia, arising without any demonstrable causal factor, strongly suggest the existence of individual predisposition. This explains also the phenomenon that after healing new lesions may develop in another site. We nevertheless accept the conclusion drawn by Vándor (1969) from his studies of a large group of patients that well-planned excision should be encouraged, as this results in healing in most cases. The detection of recurrent lesions, and thereby the prevention of further precancerosis, is a matter of regular screening, the importance of which has long been recognized and emphasized by ourselves as well as others.

Radiation therapy has usually been employed only in neoplastic lesions. Verrucous leukoplakia was once believed to respond well to irradiation (Miescher 1943), but later observations failed to substantiate this finding. Among those who have investigated the radiation therapy of oral leukoplakia only Tentchov and Andrejev (1956) have unequivocally advocated it. They attributed the failure of previous attempts at radiation therapy to the use of too low doses which give rise to mucosal inflammation and superficial erosions which are liable to malignant transformation. They therefore preferred the contact irradiation which, by causing an inflammation that also involved the deeper layers, brought about the shedding of the entire, altered epithelium. They treated 17 patients with a total dose of 5,000–8,000 r in several exposures, and achieved complete healing without relapse in each case. Salis-Samaden (1965) and Baroncelli and Questa (1965) recommended the use of a radistrontium applicator instead of contact irradiation. In Hungary, Szodoray (1963) and Szodoray and Szabó (1972) reported good therapeutic results from contact irradiation of labial leukoplakias. Fuchihata and Campas (1972) used the Dermopan apparatus with success in the treatment of labial leukoplakia. Vándor (1969) opposed the radiation therapy of oral leukoplakias on the grounds that it might cause critical changes in epithelium which is already liable to a malignant transformation, and therefore promote rather than prevent cancer development. We ourselves did not use radiation therapy in the treatment of leukoplakia.

The therapeutic results obtained in the group of 520 patients in the present study are summarized in Table 61.

In most cases, elimination of etiological factors, with or without simultaneous conservative treatment, resulted in healing or improvement. Some lesions were, however, refractory and some even showed malignant transformation (see Figs 36 and 38). *The percentage of healed and improved cases (70.6 and 27.7%, respectively) were highest among those treated surgically when causal factors could also be eliminated* (see Figs 40–42 and 40–49 as well as colour photo 8).

Mathematical–statistical analysis revealed a highly significant correlation ($p < 0.001$) between the elimination of etiological factors and healing or improvement of leukoplakia. It should be noted that the proportion of healed or improved cases, irrespective of conservative or even surgical treatment, was negligible among patients who did not collaborate in the elimination of the etiological factors, such as smoking, and ill-fitting prostheses. Spread of the lesion and cancer development was most frequent in this uncooperative group.

In our analysis of the response to treatment in relation to clinical type, we found that *healing or improvement were most frequent in the simple leukoplakias* (Table 62). No cancers developed in this particular category—the mildest in our classification—and spread of the lesion only occurred in a single case. The proportion of healed cases was lower in the verrucous category, and the incidence of "unchanged" and "spread" lesions increased over that found in simple leukoplakias while cancer developed in 4.6% of the cases.

The proportion of healed cases was lowest in the erosive category, while spread of the lesion occurred in 21 cases and cancer development in 23 (28%).

Mathematical–statistical evaluation substantiated clinical observations in that it revealed a highly significant correlation ($p < 0.001$) between the clinical type of leukoplakia and the response to therapy.

Table 61

Therapeutic results in oral leukoplakia

Methods of treatment		Healed		Improved		Unchanged		Spread		Carcinoma		Total	
		No.	%	No.	%	No.	%	No.	%	No.	%	No.	%
Etiological factors		54	43.2	55	44.0	16	12.8	—	—	—	—	125	24.0
Eliminated	+ conservative treatment	37	38.5	33	34.3	22	23.0	—	—	4	4.2	96	18.3
	+ surgical treatment	84	70.6	33	27.7	—	—	2	1.7	—	—	119	22.8
Not eliminated	or the patient did not present for treatment	—	—	—	—	77	62.6	27	22.0	19	15.4	123	23.6
	+ conservative treatment	1	3.7	1	3.7	9	33.2	8	29.7	8	29.7	27	5.6
	+ surgical treatment	—	—	9	30.0	11	36.4	10	33.3	—	—	30	5.7
Totals		176	33.8	131	25.3	135	26.0	47	9.0	31	5.9	520	100.0

Table 62

Response of the different clinical types of leukoplakia to therapy

Clinical types	Healed		Improved		Unchanged		Spread		Carcinoma		Total	
	No.	%	No.	%	No.	%	No.	%	No.	%	No.	%
Simplex	111	41.9	79	29.9	74	27.9	1	0.3	—	—	265	51.0
Verrucous	54	31.2	39	22.5	47	27.2	25	14.5	8	4.6	173	33.2
Erosive	11	13.5	13	15.9	14	17.0	21	25.6	23	28.0	82	15.8
Totals	176	33.8	131	25.3	135	26.0	47	8.0	31	5.9	520	100.0

To summarize, our experience of the treatment of leukoplakia we derived the following principles:

1. Incipient leukoplakias that do not heal 2–3 weeks after the elimination of demonstrable etiological factors require conservative or surgical treatment.

2. Conservative treatment is applied to (*a*) large, incipient lesions with slight keratinization and (*b*) large, verrucous lesions in order to reduce their size before surgical intervention.

3. Surgical treatment is applied if conservative treatment fails to produce complete healing in 3 months at the latest. The surgical excision of large lesions is undertaken gradually, over several sessions. Biopsies are always taken in this Clinic, where facilities are available for a radical intervention if required.

4. To prevent malignant change, all patients recorded with leukoplakia, including healed cases, are summoned for re-examination at least twice every year. This is to prevent the malignant transformation of precancerous forms of leukoplakia by early intervention.

CHAPTER IX

SUMMARY

1. Of 520 patients with leukoplakia in a longitudinal study with observation periods of from 1 to 25 years (mean 8.7 years), 31 (5.9%) developed carcinoma. Among the various clinical types of leukoplakia cancer development was most frequent (28%) in erosive lesions, which can thus be regarded as precancerous in the strictest sense of the term. The incidence of malignant change was 7.2% in women and 5.5% in men.

Among the various sites, leukoplakia of the tongue had the highest incidence of malignant transformation. Analysis of the age group distribution showed a prevalence of leukoplakia between 50 and 59 years, and of oral carcinoma between 60 and 69 years. Twenty-six per cent of carcinomas developed from verrucous leukoplakia and 74% from erosive leukoplakia.

2. Investigations into the role of possible etiological factors revealed that patients with a smoking habit showed a significant quantitative increase in keratinized cells over non-smokers, as measured in a comparative cytological study of 25 patients with and without the habit. Comparative histological studies of leukoplakia in smokers and non-smokers among 345 Danish and 184 Hungarian patients revealed no significant difference between keratinization patterns, epithelial thickness, and the incidence of epithelial dysplasia and connective tissue inflammation.

3. Clinical studies of the role of mechanical factors revealed their possible etiological involvement in 31.9% of the cases. Sharp-edged, broken teeth could be incriminated with the greatest certainty in 32.6% of the cases, an unsatisfactory partial prosthesis was more frequently responsible for mechanical irritation (66.6%) than a complete one (51%). Lesions related to mechanical irritation were usually found in the buccal mucosa, less often on the alveolar ridge. The greater frequency (45%) of mechanical irritation in the group with carcinoma than in the group with plain leukoplakia indicated that this may play a major role in malignant transformation.

4. An electric potential difference between metallic restorative materials was demonstrated in 3% of cases. Clinical observations suggest that electric potential difference may promote cancer development in certain conditions when other etiological factors are also present.

5. Atrophic conditions of the oral mucosa especially of the tongue, consequent upon some chronic inflammation, predispose to the development of hyperkeratosis, fissures and, ultimately cancer. A relationship between geographic tongue and the development of leukoplakia can be excluded from the clinical–pathological study of 70 cases of migratory glossitis. From clinical observations, median rhomboid glossitis and anaemic mirror tongue (Hunter–Möller glossitis, Plummer–Vinson syndrome) may both give rise to leukoplakia or cancer, probably through the indirect involvement of endogenous factors.

6. A change in the clinical type of leukoplakia took place in 66 (12.7%) of the 520 cases in the longitudinal study. Of the three types erosive leukoplakia proved to be the most changeable, especially in labial, commissural and buccal sites. Of the etiological factors, smoking and candidiasis seemed to play some part in type transformation. It was concluded that oral leukoplakia is a dynamic rather than a static lesion.

7. Of 500 lesions identified clinically as leukoplakia, histological evidence of either carcinoma, epithelial dysplasia, or non-dysplastic hyperplasia and hyperkeratosis was obtained in 48 (9.6%), 120 (24%) and 332 (66.4%) of cases, respectively. Analysis of the histological features by clinical type within the non-malignant category without dysplasia showed that simple leukoplakia was characterized by hyperorthokeratosis, the presence of a stratum granulosum and hyperplasia, verrucous leukoplakia by addition of dyskeratosis and inflammation of the subepithelial connective tissue, and erosive leukoplakia by parakeratosis, dyskeratosis, epithelial hyperplasia and inflammation of the connective tissue. It follows that there is some correlation between the clinical and histological grades of leukoplakia.

8. Analysis of the 120 leukoplakias which showed epithelial dysplasia revealed that its incidence was highest in the erosive category, above all in lesions of the tongue and lower lip. During the longitudinal study of 68 dysplastic leukoplakias over an average observation period of 6.5 years, cancer developed in nine cases (13.2%) predominantly in lingual lesions. It was found that dysplastic leukoplakia is a histologically well-defined precancerous lesion in the strictest sense of the term.

9. Cytological studies of 250 smears showed that (*a*) keratinization was enhanced in all forms of leukoplakia, and (*b*) the keratinization pattern could be indentified by cytological means. The clinical type usually showed a correlation with the keratinization pattern, as simple leukoplakia was for the most part associated with orthokeratosis (71%), erosive leukoplakia with parakeratosis (79%), and verrucous lesions with both patterns in roughly equal proportions (48 and 39%). Signs of malignant transformation were detected at the first cytological examination in 3.5% and at re-examination in 8% of the cases. Cytological study proved to be more efficient in erosive

leukoplakia than in the other two types. Comparative cytological and histological diagnosis yielded identical result in 76.6% of the cases. False negative results were most frequent in verrucous leukoplakia (32.8%), cytological diagnosis was most efficient in erosive cases (71.9%).

10. Ultrastructural studies of 12 cases of leukoplakia showed that

(*a*) in addition to, well-defined clinical and histological features, oral leukoplakia also showed characteristic changes at the ultrastructural level, and

(*b*) the strictly precancerous, dysplastic erosive lesions show typical premalignant changes that are also present in carcinoma.

11. Stereological–morphometric examination of simple leukoplakia of the buccal mucosa and floor of the mouth revealed that quantitative alterations in cytoplasmic components associated with keratinization were identical in both sites, but were reversed in comparison to normal differentiation in oral epithelium. Comparison of stereological, histopathological and clinical criteria enabled the segregation of a subgroup within the clinical category of simple leukoplakia. The stereological–morphometric approach to the measurement of epithelial differentiation in oral leukoplakia proved to be suitable for the assessment of the keratinization characteristics.

12. Scanning electron microscopic examination of specimens from six leukoplakias and one sample of normal buccal mucosa revealed differences between the surface morphology of normal and leukoplakic cells in the superficial layers, and variation in the appearance of leukoplakia in relation to clinical type. Verrucous leukoplakia characteristically showed the presence of many keratinized cells, while erosive leukoplakia exhibited disruption of the intercellular junctions and, in dysplastic cases, an atypical shape and arrangement of the cytoplasmic processes of superficial epithelial cells.

13. The differential diagnosis of oral leukoplakia includes lichen oris, leukoedema exfoliativum mucosae oris (white sponge naevus), and morsicatio buccarum et labiorum (cheek-biting). Of 326 patients with oral lichen seen in our Department 62.5% were women, most of them 40–69 years old. Oral lichen caused symptoms in 90% of the cases, and psychological stress seemed to play an important role in its etiology. The clinical type most frequently seen in our material was reticular lichen which, along with the erosive type, was less frequently associated with cutaneous symptoms than the other types. Of the patients with oral lichen 274 were available for longitudinal study over periods of from 1 to 10 years, on average 3 years. Only a single patient (0.4%) developed carcinoma.

14. Among 520 patients with oral leukoplakia and 326 with oral lichen, a total 846 cases, 27 (3.2%) showed co-existence of the two lesions within an average observation period of 5.8 years. 51.4% of the co-existent lesions were on the buccal mucosa and 21.6% on the tongue. Cancer developed in two

cases, indicating that the co-existent lesions constitute a more significant cancer hazard than either alone.

15. Clinical observation of 45 cases of leukoedema exfoliativum mucosae oris (white sponge naevus) showed that this condition chiefly affects young patients, usually with a familial incidence, and that the lesions appear exclusively in the mobile parts of the oral mucosa. This condition was more or less unresponsive to therapy, but showed neither malignant nor pre-malignant transformation during very long periods of observation. Histological and cytological studies both indicated a disturbance in keratinization characterized by faulty desquamation and a consequent accumulation of superficial parakeratotic cells.

16. Electron microscopic examination of 13 lesions of white sponge naevus revealed an abnormal arrangement of tonofilaments in comparison to normal epithelium. Neither tonofibrils nor keratohyaline granules were formed, but Odland bodies were more numerous than normal and their contents were not released into the intercellular space. Suppression of epithelial desquamations accounted for the clinical and histological pictures of epithelial hyperplasia through the accumulation of superficial cells.

17. Clinical observation of morsicatio buccarum et labiorum indicated a prevalence in the younger age groups. The main reason for adopting the habit of cheek-biting was psychological instability. Histologically reactive-epithelial hyperplasia was found. The diagnostic differentiation of the cheek-biting lesion from oral leukoplakia is easily achieved because of well-defined clinical and histological features.

18. Evaluation of the therapeutic experiences in 520 cases of oral leukoplakia has shown that surgical removal of the lesion after elimination of the etiological factors is the most efficient therapeutic approach. Among the clinical types simple leukoplakia was most responsive to conservative therapy, while a substantial number of erosive lesions showed progression or malignant change despite treatment. It has been established as a basic principle that if the elimination of etiological factors and/or conservative treatment do not result in healing of the lesion within three months at the latest, its surgical removal should be contemplated. Regular medical supervision of patients with leukoplakia at six monthly intervals is imperative even in healed cases.

REFERENCES

ALBRIGHT, J. T. (1960): Electron microscope studies of keratinization as observed in gingiva and cheek mucosa. In: The metabolism of oral tissues. *Ann. N. Y., Acad. Sci.* **85**, 351–361.

ALLMEN, G. (1978): Leukoplakie und Präkanzerose. *Schweiz. Mschr. Zahnheilk.* **87**, 310–312.

ALSHANETSKY, A. S. (1970): *cit.* Lentrodt, T. and Luhr, H. G. In: *Dtsch. Zahnärztl. Z.* **25**, 1113–1118.

AMBROSE, E. J. and ELLISON, M. (1968): Studies of specific properties of tumour cell membranes using stereoscan microscopy. *Eur. J. Cancer* **4**, 459–462.

ANASTASSOV, K. and CHPATOV, C. (1967): Du rapport étiologique entre la leucoplasie, la syphilis et le cancer de la cavité buccale. *Rev. Fr. Odontostomat.* **14**, 195–214.

ANDREASEN, J. O. (1968*a*): Oral lichen planus. *Oral Surg.* **25**, 31–42.

ANDREASEN, J. O. (1968*b*): Oral lichen planus. Oral Surg. **25**, 158–166.

ANDREASEN, J. O. and PINDBORG, J. J. (1963): Cancerudvikling und oral lichen planus. *Nord. Med.* **70**, 861–866.

ASH, C. L. (1962): Oral cancer: a twenty-five year study. *Am. J. Roentgenol.* **87**, 417–422.

ATKINSON, L., CHESTER, I. C., SMITH, F. G. and TEN SELDAM, REJ (1964): Oral cancer in New Guinea. A study in demography and etiology. *Cancer* **17**, 1289–1298.

AXELL, T. (1975): A preliminary report on prevalences of oral mucosal lesions in a Swedish population. *Community Dent. Oral Epidemiol.* **3**, 143–145.

AYRE, W. B. (1957): The cytology of oral smears. *Pan-Amer. Cancer Cytol. Cong. Miami Beach* 1957.

BAKÁCS T. (1962): Histological evaluation of leukoplakia from point of view of prevention. *Fogorv. Sz.* **55**, 8–14.

BALBAN, S. (1963): Leukoplakia hypercholesterinica oder electrogalvanica. *Z. Hautkr.* **54**, 481.

BALENDRA, W. (1949): The effect of betel chewing on the dental and oral tissues and its possible relationship to buccal carcinoma. *Br. Dent. J.* **87**, 83–86.

BALOGH, K. (1956): Clinical pathology of oral carcinoma. *Orv. Hetil.* **97**, 1093–1099.

BALOGH, K. and HUSZÁR, GY. (1962): Gerostomatological examination of gypsies. *Anthropol. Közl.* **6**, 7–8.

BALOGH, K. and LELKES K. (1965): *The Tongue.* Medicina, Budapest, pp. 95–97.

BÁNÓCZY, J. (1958): Cytological examination of normal oral mucosa. *Fogorv. Sz.* **51**, 309–315.

BÁNÓCZY, J. (1960*a*): Beiträge zur zytologischen Untersuchung der normalen Mundschleimhaut. *Dtsch. Stomat.* **10**, 486–493.

BÁNÓCZY, J. (1960*b*): Comparative exfoliative cytology of cancerous and precancerous lesions (leukoplakia, lichen) of the oral mucosa. *Acta Unio Internat. Cancer* **2,** 394–397.

BÁNÓCZY, J. (1961*a*): Cytological examinations of oral carcinoma and precarcinoma. *Magy. Onkol.* **5,** 19–25.

BÁNÓCZY, J. (1961*b*): Zytologische Untersuchungen bei karzinomatösen und präkarzinomatösen Erkrankungen der Mundschleimhaut. *Dtsch. Stomatol.* **11,** 92–97.

BÁNÓCZY, J. (1962): Observations sur l'altération de la cornification de la muqueuse buccale sous l'influence du tabac. *Bull. Group. Int. Rech. Sci.* **5,** 545–553.

BÁNÓCZY, J. (1964): Treatment of leukoplakia. *Fogorv. Sz.* **57,** 1–5.

BÁNÓCZY, J. (1965*a*): Treatment of leukoplakia preventing malignancy. *Fogorv. Sz.* **58,** 183–186.

BÁNÓCZY, J. (1965*b*): Die Therapie der Leukoplakie. *Dtsch. Stomatol.* **15,** 736–742.

BÁNÓCZY, J. (1968*a*): *Examination of keratinization of oral mucosa in physiological and pathological circumstances.* Thesis, Budapest.

BÁNÓCZY, J. (1968*b*): Cytological examinations of oral leukoplakia. *Magy. Onkol.* **12,** 221–226.

BÁNÓCZY, J. (1969*a*): Exfoliative cytological changes in oral leukoplakias. *J. Dent. Res.* **48,** 17–21.

BÁNÓCZY, J. (1969*b*): La citologia exfoliativa en las lesiones orales praecancerosas. *Rev. Assoc. Odont. Argent.* **57,** 149–154.

BÁNÓCZY, J. (1970): Clinical application of oral cytology. *Magy. Onkol.* **14,** 11–14.

BÁNÓCZY, J. (1971): Cytological study of the keratinization pattern in oral leukoplakia. *J. Dent. Res.* **50,** 1562–1566.

BÁNÓCZY, J. (1972): Zytologie der Mundhöhle. *Zahnärztl. Praxis* **23,** 124–126.

BÁNÓCZY, J. (1974): Injuries on the oral mucosa caused by prosthesis. *Fogorv. Sz.* **67,** 257–260.

BÁNÓCZY, J. (1975): Der gegenwärtige Stand der Zytologie in der Stomatologie. *Stomat. DDR* **25,** 461–469.

BÁNÓCZY, J. (1976): Exfoliative cytologic examinations in the early diagnosis of oral cancer. *Int. Dent. J.* **26,** 397–400.

BÁNÓCZY, J. (1977): Follow-up studies in oral leukoplakia. *J. Max.-Fac. Surg.* **5,** 69–75.

BÁNÓCZY, J. and CSIBA, Á. (1970): Comparative study of the clinical picture and histopathologic structure of oral leukoplakia. *Fogorv. Sz.* **63,** 65–72.

BÁNÓCZY, J. and CSIBA, Á. (1972): Comparative study of the clinical picture and histopathologic structure of oral leukoplakia. *Cancer* **29,** 1230–1234.

BÁNÓCZY, J. and CSIBA, Á. (1976*a*): Occurrence of epithelial dysplasia in oral leukoplakia. *Magy. Onkol.* **4,** 243–249.

BÁNÓCZY, J. and CSIBA, Á. (1976*b*): Occurrence of epithelial dysplasia in oral leukoplakia. *Oral Surg.* **42,** 766–774.

BÁNÓCZY, J. and RIGÓ, O. (1976): Comparative cytologic and histologic studies in oral leukoplakia. *Acta Cytol. (Baltimore)* **20,** 308–312.

BÁNÓCZY, J. and SUGÁR, L. (1968*a*): Leukoedema exfoliativum mucosae oris. *Dtsch. Zahnärztl. Z.* **23,** 478–484.

BÁNÓCZY, J. and SUGÁR, L. (1968*b*): Control results of patients with leukoplakia. *Fogorv. Sz.* **61,** 116–123.

BÁNÓCZY, J. and SUGÁR, L. (1972): Longitudinal studies in oral leukoplakias. *J. Oral Path.* **1,** 265–272.

Bánóczy, J. and Sugár, L. (1975): Progressive and regressive changes in Hungarian oral leukoplakias in the course of longitudinal studies. *Community Dent. Oral Epidemiol.* **3**, 194–197.
Bánóczy, J. and Török, O. (1972): L'effet de la vitamine A sur les cultures de tissues préparées à partir de la muqueuse buccale humaine leucoplasique. *Bull. Group. Int. Rech. Sci. Stomatol.* **15**, 117–136.
Bánóczy, J., Juhász, J. and Albrecht, M. (1978): Ultrastructure of different clinical forms of oral leukoplakia *J. Oral Pathol.* **9**, 41–53.
Bánóczy, J., Klein-Szántó, A. and Schroeder, H. (1977): Morphometric examination of oral leukoplakia simplex. *Morphol. Igazságügyi Orv. Sz.* **17**, 18–25.
Bánóczy, J., Kövesi, Gy. and Albrecht, M. (1979): Untersuchung des gemeinsamen Vork ommens von Leukoplakie und Lichen der Mundschleimhaut. *Acta Chir. Max. Fac.* **4**, 271–275.
Bánóczy, J., Lapis, K. and Albrecht, M. (1980): Scanning electronmicroscopic study of oral leukoplakia. *J. Oral Pathol.* **9**, 145–154.
Bánóczy, J., Radnai, T. and Reményi, I. (1969): Methodological experiences based on stomatooncological examinations made in the population of Dunakeszi and Felsőgöd. *Fogorv. Sz.* **62**, 118–122.
Bánóczy, J., Rigó, O. and Gábor, I. (1974): Comparative cytologic and histologic studies in oral leukoplakia. *Fogorv. Sz.* **67**, 97–101.
Bánóczy, J., Roed-Petersen, B., Pindborg, J. J. and Inovay, J. (1979): Clinical and histologic studies on electrogalvanically induced oral white lesions. *Oral Surg.* **48**, 319–323.
Bánóczy, J., Sugár, L. and Frithiof, I. (1973): White sponge nevus: Leukoedema exfoliativum mucosae oris. *Sved. Dent. J.* **66**, 481–493.
Bánóczy, J., Szabó, L. and Csiba, Á. (1974): Data on clinicopathology of glossitis migrans. *Fogorv. Sz.* **67**, 33–37.
Bánóczy, J., Szabó, L. and Csiba, Á. (1975): Migratory glossitis. A clinical-histological review of seventy cases. *Oral Surg.* **39**, 113–121.
Baroncelli, G. and Questa, L. (1965): Il problema terapeutica della leucoplasia del cavo orale. *Riv. Ital. Stomatol.* **20**, 1290–1299.
Barucchi, G. B., Ferrando, O. and Mangiante, P. (1963): Indagine al microscopio elettronico sull'epitelio della mucosa orale normale, leucoplasica e carcinomatosa: aspetti ultramicroscopici dell'epitelio di mucosa geniens leucoplasica. *Riv. Ital. Stomatol.* **18**, 1697–1969.
Basset, B. B. and Pacher, I. (1965): Response of isolated lysosomes to Vitamin A. *J. Cell Biol.* **27**, 448–450.
Baughman, R. A. and Charleston, S. L. (1971): Median rhomboid glossitis. A developmental anomaly? *Oral Surg.* **31**, 56–65.
Bernimoulin, J. P. and Schroeder, H. E. (1977): Quantitative electron microscopic analysis of the epithelium of normal human alveolar mucosa. *Cell Tiss. Res.* **180**, 383–401.
Bernstein, H. F. and Lewin, R. W. (1959): White sponge nevus. *Oral Surg.* **10**, 1200–1212.
Bodart, L. (1968): Les cancers multiples de la cavité buccale. *Acta Stomatol. Belg.* **65**, 295–340.
Borello, E. D., de Geiler, L. E. and Poex, A. (1972): Median rhomboid glossitis. *Oral Res. Abstracts* **7**, 419.
Boyle, P. E. (1954): Differential diagnosis of soft tissue lesions of the mouth with a discussion of biopsy procedures. *Oral Surg.* **7**, 507–514.

BRADLEY, J. L. (1956): Leukoplakia of the lower lip. *Oral Surg.* **9**, 776–785.

BRANDES, D. and ANTON, C. (1966): Lysosomes in cellular lytic processes. III. Electron histochemical changes in mammary tumours after treatment with Cytoxan and vitamin A. *Lab. Invest.* **15**, 987–1006.

BREDY, E. (1955): Beitrag zur Kenntnis der Leukoplakie der Mundhöhle. *Dtsch. Stomatol.* **5**, 88–96.

BREITNER, J. (1950): Glossitis rhomboica mediana. *Münch. Med. Wschr.* **92**, 350.

BROCQ, L. and PAUTRIER, L. M. (1914–15): Glossite losangique médiane de la face dorsale de la langue. *Ann. Derm. Syph. (Paris)* **5**, 1–5.

BRODY, I. (1960): The ultrastructure of the tonofibrils in the keratinization process of normal human epidermis. *J. Ultrastruct. Res.* **4**, 264–297.

BROWN, C. B. (1962): Treatment of leukoplakia of the lip. Report of a case. *J. Oral Surg.* **20**, 77–79.

BROWNE, W. G., IZATT, M. M. and RENWICK, J. H. (1969): White sponge nevus of the mucosa: Clinical and linkage data. *Ann. Hum. Genet.* **32**, 271–281.

BRUNNER, K. (1975): Therapie mit Vitamin A-Verbindungen. *Arbeitssitzung des Deutsch-Öst. Schweiz. Arbeitskreises für Tumoren im Kiefer-Gesichtsbereich. Basel, 1975. 20–21. XI.*

BRUSZT, P. (1962*a*): Stomato-oncological screening examinations in the region of Baja and Bácsalmás. *Magy. Onkol.* **6**, 28–33.

BRUSZT, P. (1962*b*): Stomato-onkologische Reihenuntersuchungen in sieben Gemeinden Südungarns. *Schweiz. Mschr. Zahnheilk.* **72**, 758–766.

BURKHARDT, A. (1980): *Der Mundhöhlenkrebs und seine Vorstadien.* Fischer, Stuttgart–New York, pp. 60–92.

BURKHARDT, A. and SEIFERT, G. (1977): Morphologische Klassifikation der oralen Leukoplakien. *Dtsch. Med. Wschr.* **102**, 223–229.

CAHN, L. R., EISENBUD, L. and BLAKE, M. (1961): Histochemical analyses of white lesions of the mouth. *Oral Surg.* **14**, 596–602.

CALONIUS, P. E. B. (1961): A cytological study on the variation of keratinization on the normal oral mucosa of young males. *Suom. Hammaslääk, toim.* **57**, 163.

CANNON, A. B. (1935): White sponge nevus of the mucosa (naevus spongiosus albus mucosae). *Arch. Derm. Syph.* **31**, 365–370.

CAWSON, R. A. (1966): Chronic oral candidiasis and leukoplakia. *Oral Surg.* **22**, 582–591.

CAWSON, R. A. (1975): Premalignant lesions in the mouth. *Br. Med. Bull.* **31**, 164–168.

CARSON, R. A. and BINNIE, W. H. (1980): Candida leukoplakia and carcinoma: a possible relationship. In: *Oral Premalignancy.* Ed by J. C. Mackenzie, E. Dabelsteen and Ch. A. Squier. University of Iowa Press, Iowa City, pp. 59–66.

CERNÉA, P., KUFFER, R. and BROCHERIOU, C. (1971*a*): L'épithélioma sur lichen plan buccal (à propos de 40 nouvelles observations). *Actual Odontostomatol.* **96**, 473–490.

CERNÉA, P., GUILBERT, F. and KUFFER, R. (1971*b*): Épithéliomas évoluant sur lichen plan buccal. Quarante nouvelles observations. *J. Fr. Otorhinolaringol.* **20**, 1015–1017.

CHASE, H. (1879): Oral electricity. *D. Cosmos* **21**, 205–207.

CHOSACK, A., ZADIK, L. and EIDELMAN, E. (1974): The prevalence of scrotal tongue and geographic tongue in 70,359 Israeli schoolchildren. *Community Dent. Oral Epidemiol.* **2**, 235–257.

CLEMMESEN, J. (1965): *Statistical Studies in the Etiology of Malignant Neoplasms.* Munksgaard, Kobenhavn, pp. 93–95.

COOKE, B. E. D. (1954): The oral manifestation of lichen planus: 50 cases. *Br. Dent. J.* **96**, 1–9.

COOKE, B. E. D. (1956): Leukoplakia buccalis and oral epithelial naevi. *Br. J. Derm.* **68,** 151–174.
COOKE, B. E. D. (1962): Median rhomboid glossitis and benign glossitis migrans. *Br. Dent. J.* **112,** 389–393.
COOKE, B. E. D. (1967): Keratinizing lesions affecting the oral mucosa. *Proc. Roy. Soc. Med.* **60,** 819–822.
COOKE, B. E. D. (1975): Oral leukoplakia: enigma? *Proc. Roy. Soc. Med.* **68,** 337–341.
COOKE, B. E. D. and MORGAN, J. (1959): Oral epithelial naevi. *Br. J. Derm.* **11,** 134–138.
DABELSTEEN, E. (1980): Introduction to tumor immunology and immunological aspects of oral premalignant lesions, In: *Oral Premalignancy.* Ed. by J. C. Mackenzie, E. Dabelsteen and Ch. A. Squier. University of Iowa Press, Iowa City, pp. 269–285.
DABELSTEEN, E., ROED-PETERSEN, B., SMITH, J. and PINDBORG, J. J. (1971): The limitations of exfoliative cytology for the detection of epithelial atypia in oral leukoplakias. *Br. J. Cancer* **25,** 21–24.
DAFTARY, D. K., METHA, F. S., GUPTA, P. C. and PINDBORG, J. J. (1972): The presence of Candida in 723 oral leukoplakias among Indian villagers. *Scand. J. Dent. Res.* **80,** 75–79.
DARLING, O. E. and FLETCHER, J. P. (1958): Familiar white folded gingivo-stomatitis **87,** 827–828.
DAWSON, T. A. J. (1969): Microscopic appearance of geographic tongue. *Br. J. Derm.* **87,** 827–828.
DECHAUME, M. and PAYEN, J. (1969): Les lésions anatomo-pathologiques du lichen plan buccal d'après 115 observations. *Rev. Stomat.* **70,** 47–52.
DECHAUME, M., PAYEN, J. and HAYE, K. (1958): Glossitis losangique médiane de Brocq et Pautrier. *Rev. Stomatol.* **59,** 289–304.
DECHAUME, M., PAYEN, J. and PIRIOU, H. (1957): Le lichen plan isolé de la muqueuse buccale. Considérations anatomo-cliniques d'après 50 observations dont 30 avec examen histologique. *Presse Méd.* **94,** 2133–2145.
DELESSE, M. A. (1847): Procédé mécanique pour déterminer la composition des roches. *C. R. Acad. Sci. (Paris)* **25,** 544–548.
DENIER, L. (1955): La pathologie engendrée par le galvanisme buccal, un micropyle permanent. *Ann. Odonto-stomatol. (Lyon)* **12,** 211–213.
DEPAOLI, M. (1964): Rilievi clinico-statistici sul lichen ruber planus. *Minerva Dermatol.* **39,** 166–171.
DINGLE, J. T. and LUCY, J. A. (1965): Vitamin A, carotenoids and cell function. *Biol. Rev.* **40,** 442–444.
DINGLE, J. T., SHERMAN, I. M. and MOORE, T. (1966): Nutrition and lysosomal activity. *Biochem. J.* **28,** 476–484.
EHRL, P. A. (1980): Klinische Untersuchung eines aromatischen Retinoids (Ro-10-9359) zur Behandlung oraler Hyperkeratosen. *Dtsch. Zahnärztl. Z.* **35,** 554–558.
EINHORN, J. and WERSÄLL, J. (1967): Incidence of oral carcinoma in patients with leukoplakia of the oral mucosa. *Cancer* **20,** 2189–2193.
EL-LABBAN, N. G. and KRAMER, I. R. H. (1974*a*): On the so-called microgranules in the nonkeratinized buccal epithelium. *J. Ultrastruct. Res.* **48,** 377–387.
EL-LABBAN, N. G. and KRAMER, I. R. H. (1974*b*): On the so-called membrane-coating granules in human oral epithelium. *J. Dent. Res.* **53,** 1071–1072.
EL-LABBAN, N. G. and KRAMER, I. R. H. (1975): Light and electron microscopic study of liquefaction degeneration in oral lichen planus. *Arch. Oral Biol.* **20,** 653–657.

El-Labban, N. G., Lucas, R. B. and Kramer, I. R. H. (1971): The mitotic values for the epithelium in oral keratoses and lichen planus. *Br. J. Cancer* **25**, 411–416.
Engels, A., Karczag, C., Sturza, T. and Schwarzkopf, A. (1958): Consideratii anatomo-clinice asupra leucoplasiei bucale. *Stomatologia (Bucureşti)* **5**, 289–291.
Engelstad, R. B. (1941): Glossitis rhombica mediana. *Strahlentherapie.* **70**, 692–698.
Everett, F. G. and Noyes, H. J. (1963): White folded gingivostomatosis. *J. Periodontol.* **24**, 32–41.
Farman, A. G. (1976*a*): Tongue fissure. A classification and comparative prevalence study among 825 European Caucasian and 605 Xhosa Negro school children. *J. Biol. Buccale* **4**, 349–364.
Farman, A. G. (1976*b*): Atrophic lesions of the tongue: A prevalence study among 175 diabetic patients. *J. Oral Path.* **5**, 255–264.
Farman, A. G. and Lawton, F. E. (1966): *Stone's Oral and Dental Diseases.* Livingstone, Edinburgh, p. 696.
Farman, A. G. and Nutt, G. (1976): Oral candida, debilitating disease and atrophic lesions of the tongue. *J.Biol. Buccale* **4**, 203–216.
Farman, A. G., van Wyk, C. W., Salz, J. and Dreyer, W. P. (1975): Central papillary atrophy of the tongue. *Proc. Ninth Ann. Congr. of the South Afr. Div. Int. Ass. for Dent. Res. Johannesburg.* Abstr. p. 1.
Farman, A. G., van Wyk, C. W., Salz, J., Hugo, M. and Dreyer, W. P. (1977): Central papillary atrophy of the tongue. *Oral Surg.* **43**, 48–58.
Fasske, E. and Morgenroth, K. (1964): *Pathologische Histologie der Mundhöhle.* Hirzel, Leipzig. p. 53.
Fasske, E. and Themann, H. (1958): Über das Deckepithel der menschlichen Mundschleimhaut. *Zellforschung* **49**, 447–463.
Fasske, E , Hahn, W., Morgenroth, K. and Themann, H. (1958): Die Leukoplakie der menschlichen Mundschleimhaut. *Mitteilungsdienst* **2**, 7–24.
Fasske, E., Hahn, E., Morgenroth, K. and Themann, H. (1959*a*): Die Früherkennung des Carcinomas in der Mundhöhle. *Dtsch. Zahnärztl. Z.* **14**, 251–253.
Fasske, E., Hahn, W., Morgenroth, K. and Themann, K. (1959*b*): Die formale und kausale Genese der Leukoplakia oris. *Z. Haut-Kr.* **26**, 339–347.
Fox, C. (1884): On the circinate eruption of the tongue. *Lancet* **1**, 842–844.
Fraska, J. M. and Parks, V. R. (1965): A routine technique for double staining ultrathin sections using uranyl and lead salts. *J. Cell Biol.* **25**, 157–163.
Freedman, G. L., Hooley, J. R. and Redman, R. S. (1967): Median rhomboid glossitis. An atypical variant. *Oral Surg.* **24**, 621–622.
Freihofer, H. P. (1978): Das klinische Bild der Präkanzerose. *Schweiz. Mschr. Zahnheilk.* **88**. 486–496.
Frithiof, L. (1963): Electron microscopical observations on hyperkeratinization in oral mucosa. *Acta Otolaryngol. (Suppl.) (Stockh.)* **188**, 423–429.
Frithiof, L. (1969): Ultrastructure of the basement membrane in normal and hyperplastic human oral epithelium compared with that in preinvasive and invasive carcinoma. *Acta Pathol. Microbiol. Scand.* **200**, 1–63.
Frithiof, L. (1970): Ultrastructural changes in the plasma membrane in human oral epithelium. *J. Ultrastruct. Res.* **32**, 1–17.
Frithiof, L. (1971): Electron microscopic observations on structures related to the epithelial basement membrane in squamous cell carcinoma. *Acta Otolaryngol. (Stockh.)* **71**, 323–334.
Frithiof, L. (1972): Cytoplasmic processes in normal and in malignant oral epithelium. *Acta Otolaryngol. (Stockh.)* **74**, 212–229.

Frithiof, L. and Bánóczy, J. (1976a): White sponge nevus (leukoedema exfoliativum mucosae oris). Ultrastructural observations. *Oral Surg.* **41**, 607–622.

Frithiof, L. and Bánóczy, J. (1976b): Electronmicroscopical observations in clinical picture of leukoedema exfoliativum mucosae oris (white sponge nevus). *Morphol. Igazságügyi Orv. Sz.* **16**, 31–37.

Frithiof, L. and Wersäll, J. (1965): A highly ordered structure in keratinizing human oral epithelium. *J. Ultrastruc. Res.* **12**, 371–379.

Frithiof, L. and Wersäll, J. (1966): Phospholipid-like granules in keratinizing epithelium. *Swedish Canc. Soc., Yearbook* **4**, 88–91.

Frithiof, L. and Wersäll, J. (1968): Some electron microscopic observations on the basement membrane in oral precancerous and cancerous lesions. In: *"Oral Surg." Congress Transactions*. Ed. by E., Husted and E. Hjorting-Hansen. Munksgaard, Copenhagen, pp. 40–43.

Frykholm, O., Frithiof, L., Fernström, B., Moberger, G., Blohm, S. and Björn, E. (1969): Allergy to copper derived from dental alloys as a possible cause of oral lesions of lichen planus. *Acta Derm. Venereol. (Stockh.)* **49**, 268–281.

Fuchihata, E. and Campas, C. A. (1972): Radiotherapy of carcinoma developed from leukoplakia. *Oral. Surg.* **33**, 137–143.

Fulling, H. J. (1973): Cancer development in oral lichen planus. A follow-up study of 327 patients. *Arch. Dermatol.* **108**, 667–669.

Fülöp, É. (1957): Lichen ruber planus cases healed by ACTH-treatment. *Bőrgyógy. Venereol. Sz.* **44**, 151–154.

Gangadharan, P. and Paymaster, J. C. (1971): Leukoplakia — an epidemiologic study of 1,504 cases observed at the Tata Memorial Hospital, Bombay, India. *Br. J. Cancer* **25**, 657–668.

Gardner, V. F. (1964): An investigation of the use of exfoliative cytology in the diagnosis of malignant lesions of the oral cavity. *Acta Cytol. (Baltimore)* **8**, 436–451.

Gaston, K. (1969): *cit.* by Dawson.

Gaudy, D. T. (1952): Nevus spongiosus albus mucosae. *Tex. Med.* **48**, 145.

Gautier, V. (1881): De la desquamation épithéliale de la langue. *Rev. Méd. Suisse Romande* **1**, 589–607.

Gemell, R. T. and Chapman, R. E. (1971): Formation and breakdown of the inner root sheath and features of the pilary canal epithelium in the wool follicle. *J. Ultrastruct. Res.* **36**, 355–366.

Gerry, R. G., Smith, S. T. and Calton, M. L. (1952): The oral characteristics of Guamanians including the effects of betel chewing on the oral tissues. *Oral Surg.* **5**, 762–781, 894, 994, 1004–1011.

Gigliardi, M. R., Mongini, F. and Mela, F. (1966): Rilievi su una casistica di lesioni cosidette leucoplasiche del cavo orale. *Il Cancero (Torino)* **19**, 567–586.

Gombos, F. Caruso, F., Galantuomo, P. and Buonaiuto, C. (1973): Quadri di patologia orale: il lichen ruber planus della mucosa orale. *Riv. Ital. Stomacol.* **28**, 237–258.

Gombos, F., Caruso, F. and Matarasso, S. (1974): Quadri di patologia orale: le leucoplasie della mucosa orale. *Riv. Ital. Stomacol.* **29**, 465–482.

Greither, A. (1955): *Dermatologie der Mundhöhle und der Mundumgebung*. Thieme, Stuttgart, pp. 18–19.

Greither, A. (1970): Leukoplakien der Lippen und der Mundschleimhaut. *Dtsch. Zahnärztl. Z.* **25**, 961–973.

Grinspan, T., Diaz, J., Abulafia, J., Villapol, L., Schneidermann, J., Palese, D.

and Bedrichesky, R. (1966): Notre expérience sur le lichen ruber planus de la muqueuse buccale. *Ann. Derm. Syph.* **93**, 531–542.
Gupta, P. C., Mehta, F. S., Daftary, D. K., Pindborg, J. J., Bhonsle, R. B., Jainawalla, P. N., Sinor, P. N., Pitkar, P. N., Murti, P. R., Irani, R. R., Shah, H. T., Kadam, P. M., Iyer, K. S. S., Iyer, H. M., Hegde, G. K., Chandrashekar, G. K., Shroff, B. C., Sahiar, B. E. and Mehta, M. N. (1980): Incidence rates of oral cancer and natural history of oral precancerous lesions in a 10-year follow-up study of Indian villagers. *Community Dent. Oral Epidemiol.* **8**, 287–333.
Hahn, W. (1962*a*): Altersveränderungen der Mundschleimhaut. *Dtsch. Zahnärztebl.* **15**, 410–416.
Hahn, W. (1962*b*): Vergleichende histologische und exfoliativcytologische Untersuchungen in Leukoplakien der Mundschleimhaut. *Dtsch. Zahnärztebl.* **16**. 698–700.
Hahn, W. and Lange, D. (1967): Histo- und zytochemische Reaktionen bei der Untersuchung von Mundschleimhauterkrankungen. *Zahn, Mund Kieferheilk.* **49**, 396–409.
Hahn, W., Morgenroth, K. and Themann, H. (1961): Precancerous changes in the oral cavity. *Int. Dent. J.* **11**, 343–362.
Haim, G. (1964): Elektronenmikroskopische Untersuchungen pathologischer Verhornungsvorgänge im Epithel der Mundschleimhaut. *Stoma* **17**, 292–306.
Hallopeau, H. (1910): Sur un cas de lichen de Wilson gingival avec néoplasie voisine dans la région maxillaire. *Bull. Soc. Fr. Derm. Syph.* **17**, 32.
Halperin, V., Kolas, S., Jefferies, K. P., Huddleston, S. O. and Robinson, H. B. C. (1953): Occurrence of Fordyce spots, benign migratory glossitis, median rhomboid glossitis and fissured tongue in 2,478 dental patients. *Oral Surg.* **6**, 1072–1077.
Hammer, B. and Schroeder, H. E. (1977): Stereologic system an on/off-line computer program for analysing oral epithelia, based on a model of stratification. *Arch. Oral Biol.* **22**, 337–341.
Hansen, L. (1959): Diagnosis of oral keratotic lesions. *J. Oral Surg.* **17**, 60–66.
Hansen, U. (1942): Glossitis rhombica mediana. *Nord. Med. (Stockh.)* **220**, 1940, Ref. nach *Zbl. Hals- Nas-, Ohrenheilk.* **35**, 49.
Hashimoto, K. (1971): Fine structure of horny cells of the vermilion border of the lip compared with skin. *Arch. Oral Biol.* **16**, 397–410.
Hashimoto, K., DiBella, R. J. and Shklar, G. (1966): Electron microscopic studies of the normal human buccal mucosa. *J. Invest. Derm.* **47**, 512–525.
Hashimoto, K., DiBella, R. J., Tarnowsky, W. M. and Shklar, G. (1968): Electron microscopic studies of oral benign leukoplakia. *Oral Surg.* **25**, 901–913.
Hazen, H. H. (1935): Syphilis and skin diseases in the American Negro. *Arch. Derm. Syph.* **31**, 316–318.
Haye, K. R. and Whitehead, P. I. H. (1968): Hereditary leukokeratosis of the mucous membranes. *Br. J. Derm.* **80**, 529—533.
Haym, J. (1961): Die Praecancerose in der Mundhöhle. *Dtsch. Zahnärztl. Z.* **16**, 58–70.
Hayward, A. P. (1973): Electron microscopic observations on cell coat and membrane-coating granules of the epithelium of the hard soft palate in the rat. *Arch. Oral Biol.* **18**, 67–75.
Hellinger, M. J., Karpas, Ch. M. and Sellers, M. (1963): A clinicopathologic correlation of oral white lesions. *Oral Surg.* **16**, 1365–1376.
Hermann, D. (1963): Veränderungen der Gingiva bei Lichen planus und ihre Bezie-

hungen zur sogenannten Gingivitis desquamativa. *Dtsch. Zahnärztl. Z.* **18,** 1052–1057.

HERMANN, D. (1974): Leukoedema exfoliativum mucosae oris. *Dtsch. Zahnärztl. Z.* **29,** 38–43.

HERTZ, J. (1956): Oral precancerous lesions. *Oral Surg.* **9,** 686–695.

HETESSY, G. (1960*a*): Über Präkanzerosen der Mundhöhle. *Dtsch. Zahnärztebl.* **12,** 365–373.

HETESSY, G. (1960*b*): Oral carcinoma caused by chemical agents and chemical therapy of malignant tumours. *Fogorv. Sz.* **53,** 98–105.

HJØRTING-HANSEN, E. and HOLST, E. (1970): Morsicatio mucosae oris and suctio mucosae oris. *Scand. J. Dent. Res.* **76,** 492–499.

HOBAEK, A. (1947) Leukoplakia oris. *Acta Odontol. Scand.* **7,** 61–65.

HOLLANDER, I., PERMÁR, H. and SCHONFIELD, L. (1933): Leukoplakia of the oral mucosa. *J. Amer. Dent. Ass.* **20,** 51–56.

HORNSTEIN, O. P. (1976): *Zungenveränderungen.* Fortschr. prakt. Dermatologie und Venerologie. Vol. 8. Springer, Berlin—Heidelberg.

HORNSTEIN, O. P. (1977*a*): Leukoplakien der Mundschleimhaut. *Zbl. Haut- u. Geschlechtskrank.* **139,** 1–18.

HORNSTEIN, O. P. (1977*b*): Orale Leukoplakien. I. Klassifikation, Differentialdiagnose, ätiologische Bedingungen der Kanzerisierung, Prognose. *Dtsch. Zahnärztl. Z.* **32,** 497–505.

HORSTEIN, O. P., GRÄSSEL, R., SCHIRNER, E. and SCHELL, H. (1979): Orale Candida-Besiedlung bei Leukoplakien und Karzinömen der Mundhöhle. *Dtsch. Med. Wschr.* **104,** 1033–1036.

HYAMS, M. N. and BLOOM, O. H. (1947): Leukoplakia vulvae: its etiology and results of treatment with vitamin A. *Am. J. Obstet. Gynec.* **53,** 214.

INOVAY, J. and BÁNÓCZY, J. (1960*a*): Effets de la différence des potentiels électriques sur la muqueuse buccale provoqués par des métaux divers. *Rev. Stomatol.* **61,** 669–676.

INOVAY, J. and BÁNÓCZY, J. (1960*b*): Electrical potential differences in the aetiology of the diseases of the oral mucosa. *Fogorv. Sz.* **63,** 260–264.

INOVAY, J. and BÁNÓCZY, J. (1961): The role of electrical potential differences in the etiology of chronic diseases of the oral mucosa. *J. Dent. Res.* **40,** 884–890.

ISHIBASHI, Y. and KLINGMÜLLER, G. (1968): Erythrodermia ichthyosiformis congenita bullosa Brocq, II. Electron microscopic investigation of the basal and prickled cell layer. *Arch. Klin. Experim. Dermat.* **232,** 205–224.

JACOBS, J. B., ARAI, M., COHEN, S. M. and FRIDELL, G. H. (1976): Light and scanning electron microscopy of exfoliated bladder cells in rats fed N-(4-)5-nitro-2-furyl(-2--thiazolyl) formamide. *J. Nat. Canc. Inst.* **57,** 63–66.

JEPSEN, A. and WINTHER, J. E. (1965): Mycotic infection in oral leukoplakia. *Acta Odontol. Scand.* **23,** 239–256.

JORDAN, J. A. and WILLIAMS, A. E. (1973): Scanning electron microscopy in the study of cervical neoplasia. J. *Obstet. Gynec. Brit. Comm.* **28,** 940–946.

KAMALAMMA, M. K., PRABHU, S. R., SHETTY, J. N. and RAGHUNATHA RAO N. (1970): The white sponge nevus. *Oral Surg.* **30,** 51–54.

KARNOVSKY, M. J. (1961): Simple methods for "staining with lead" at high pH in electron microscopy. *J. Biophys. Biochem. Cytol.* **11,** 729–732.

KEMPSON, S. A. (1974): The ultrastructural classification of keratohyalin granules of the rat oral epithelium. *J. Dent. Res.* **53,** Suppl. 5. 1072.

KING, O. H. and COLEMAN, S. A. (1965): Analysis of oral exfoliative cytologic accuracy by control biopsy technique. *Acta Cytol.* **9,** 351–354.

KINNEY, R. C. and DERIFIELD, R. S. (1956): Pachydermia oralis: report of case. *J. Oral Surg.* **14**, 71–73.
KISS, GY. (1955): Etiology of leukoplakia oris. Congress of Hungarian Dermatologists 1955.
KLEIN-SZÁNTÓ, A. J. P., ANDERSEN, L. and SCHROEDER, H. E. (1976): Epithelial differentiation patterns in buccal mucosa affected by lichen planus. *Virchows Arch. (Cell Pathol.)* **22**, 245–261.
KLEIN-SZÁNTÓ, A. J. P., BÁNÓCZY, J. and SCHROEDER, H. E. (1976): Metaplastic conversion of the differentiation pattern in oral epithelia affected by leukoplakia simplex. *Pathologia Europaea* **11**, 180–210.
KLEIN-SZÁNTÓ, A. J. P. and SCHROEDER, H. E. (1977): Architecture and density of connective tissue papillae of the human oral mucosa. *J. Anat.* **123**, 93–109.
KLEISS, E. (1949): Zur Genese der Glossitis rhombica mediana. *Arch. Ohr.-Nas.-Kehlk. Heilk.* **155**, 490–496.
KNYCHALSKA-KARWAN, S. (1964): Badanie cytologiczne leukoplakii blony sliuzowej policzkow. *Chas. Stomatol. (Warszawa)* **17**, 841.
KNYCHALSKA-KARWAN, S. (1965*a*): Wplyw tytoniu ne blone sluzowa jamy ustnej. *Chas. Stomatol. (Warszawa)* **18**, 621–628.
KNYCHALSKA-KARWAN, S. (1965*b*): Ocena podzialow leukoplakii. *Chas. Stomatol. (Warsawa)* **18**, 775–781.
KNYCHALSKA-KARWAN, S. (1965*c*): Leczenie leukoplakii blony sluzowej jami ustnej. *Chas. Stomatol. (Warsawa)* **18**, 1293–1298.
KOCH, H. and SCHETTLER, D. (1973): Klinische Erfahrungen mit Vitamin A-Säure Derivaten bei der Behandlung von Leukoplakien der Mundschleimhaut. *Dtsch. Zahnärztl. Z.* **28**, 623–627.
KOCSARD, E., SCHWARZ, L., STEPHEN, B. S. and D'ABRERA, E. R. (1962): Morsicatio buccarum. *Br. J. Derm.* **74**, 545–547.
KOLLAR, J. A., FINLEY, G. W., NABERS, J., RITCHEY, B. and ORBAN, B. J. (1954): Leukoplakia *J. Amer. Dent. Ass.* **49**, 538–548.
KONSTANTINOV, A., JAVOV, S. and VATKOV, I. (1959): Contribution à la clinique et à l'histopathologie du lichen plan de la muqueuse buccale. *Izv. Otd. Biol. Med. Nauki. (Sofia)* **3**. 81–87.
KOVÁCS, GY. (1962*a*): Die moderne Diagnostik und Therapie von Präblastomatosen der Mundhöhle. *Ther. Hung.* **10**, 3/1–3.
KOVÁCS, GY. (1962*b*): *Preblastomatosis of oral cavity.* Thesis, Budapest.
KÖVESI, GY. (1973): Treatment of lichen oris with Delagil. *Bőrgyógy. Venereol. Sz.* **49**, 171–174.
KÖVESI, GY. and BÁNÓCZY, J. (1973*a*): Catamnestic follow-up of patients with lichen. *Fogorv. Sz.* **66**, 74–79.
KÖVESI, GY. and BÁNÓCZY, J. (1973*b*): Relationship between the partial denture and the hyperkeratosis of oral mucosa. *Fogorv. Sz.* **66**, 467–469.
KÖVESI, GY. and BÁNÓCZY, J. (1973*c*): Follow-up studies in oral lichen planus. *Int. J. Oral Surg.* **2**, 13–19.
KÖVESI, GY., GERA, I. and CSIBA, Á. (1975): Carcinoma developed following lichen oris. *Fogorv. Sz.* **68**, 265–268.
KRAMER, I. R. H. (1969): Praecancerous conditions of the oral mucosa. *Ann. R. Coll. Surg. Engl.* **45**, 3–19.
KRAMER, I. R. H. (1976): Precancerous lesions of the mouth. *J. Laryngol.-Otol.* **15**, 95–100.
KRAMER, I. R. H., EL-LABBAN, N. G. and LEE, K. W. (1978): The clinical features

and risk of malignant transformation in sublingual keratosis. *Br. Dent. J.* **144**, 171–180.
KRAMER, I. R. H., EL-LABBAN, N. G. and SONKODI, S. (1974): Further studies on lesions of the oral mucosa using computer-aided analyses of histological features. *Br. J. Cancer* **29**, 223–231.
KRAMER, I. R. H., LUCAS, R. B., EL-LABBAN, N. G. and LISTER L. (1970*a*): A computer aided study on the tissue changes in oral keratoses and lichen planus, and an analysis of case groupings by subjective and objective criteria. *Br. J. Cancer* **24**, 407–426.
KRAMER, I. R. H., LUCAS, R. B., EL-LABBAN, N. G. and LISTER, I. (1970*b*): The use of discriminant analysis for examining the histological features of oral keratoses and lichen planus. *Br. J. Cancer* **24**, 673–686.
KRUTCHKOFF, D. J., CUTLER, L. and LASKOWSKI, S. (1978): Oral lichen planus. *J. Oral Path.* **7**, 1–7.
KUFFER, R. (1972): Les affections précancereuses de la muqueuse buccale. *Méd. Hyg.* **30**, 669–670.
KUFFER, R. (1975): Arbeitssitzung des Deutsch. Öst. Schweiz. Arbeitskreises für Tumoren im Kiefer-und Gesichtsbereich. Basel, XI. 20–21, 1975.
KUFFER, R. and ROUCHON, C. (1967): Pour une nouvelle conception des kératoses buccales. *Actual. Odontostomatol. (Paris)* **79**, 269–293.
KUFFER, R. and BROCHERIOU, C. (1968): Notions d'actualité sur la langue géographique. *Stomatologia, Entretiens de Bichat,* 19–23.
KUFFER, R., BROCHERIOU, C. and CERNÉA, P. (1971): Exfoliatio areata linguae et mucosae oris. *Rev. Stomatol.* **72**, 109–119.
KUFFER, R. and FIORE-DONNO, G. (1977): Le carcinome intraépithélial de la muqueuse buccale et ses variantes anatomocliniques. *Rev. mens. suisse Odonto-stomatol.* **87**, 1222–1227.
KUHN, E. and RAVASZ, L. (1964): Tongue carcinoma developed following Plummer–Vinson syndrome. *Fogorv. Sz* **57**, 10–14.
KWAPIS, B. W. and GIBSON, M. J. (1956): Surgical treatment of precancerous lesions of the lip. *J. Oral Surg.* **14**, 195–198.
LAIN, E. (1933): Electrogalvanic lesions of the oral cavity produced by metallic dentures. *J. Amer. Dent. Ass.* **100**, 717–723.
LAINSON, P. A. and MACKENZIE, I. C. (1975): Cytological changes in gingiva of young smokers. *J. Dent. Res.* **54**, Suppl. Nr. 73, 63.
LANDAY, M. A. and SCHROEDER, H. E. (1976): Quantitative electron microscopic analysis of the non-keratinizing epithelium of normal human buccal mucosa. *Cell Tiss. Res.* **177**, 383–405.
LANE, J. E. (1924): Glossitis rhombica mediana. *Arch. Derm. Syph.* **9**, 547–548.
LAUFFER, J. and KUFFER, R. (1970): *Le lichen plan buccal.* Masson, Paris, pp. 82–90.
LEHNER, T. (1971): Quantitative assessment of lymphocytes and plasma cells in leukoplakia, candidiasis and lichen planus. *J. Dent. Res.* **50**. 1661–1665.
LEHNER, T., WILTON, J. M., SHILLITOE, E. J. and IVÁNYI, L. (1973): Cell-mediated immunity and antibodies to Herpes-virus hominis type 1 in oral leukoplakia and carcinoma. *Br. J. Cancer* **27**, 351–356.
LELKES, K. (1973): Significance of intermediary zones at preanodontial stage. *Fogorv. Sz.* **66**, 469–472.
LENTRODT, J. and LUHR, H. G. (1970): Diagnostische Probleme bei der Glossitis rhombica mediana. *Dtsch. Zahnärztl. Z.* **25**, 1118.

LEOPARD, P. M. and POSWILLO, D. E. (1974): Practical cryosurgery for oral lesions. *Br. Dent. J.* **136**, 185–196.

LEVIJ, I. S. and POLLIACK, A. (1968): The potentiating effect of vitamin A on 9–10 Dimetyl 1-1-2-Benzanthracene-carcinogenesis in the hamster cheek-pouch. *Cancer* **22**, 300–306.

LEWIS, B. (1955): Effect of smoking on the oral mucosa. *Oral Surg.* **8**, 1026–1033.

LOOS, H. O. and HÖRBST, L. (1934): Über das Wesen der "Glossitis rhomboica mediana". *Arch. Ohr-Nas-Kehlkheilk.* **138**, 122–132.

LÖNING, TH., BURKHARDT, A., SEIFERT, G. and GEBBERS, J. O. (1977): Zur Typisierung der Immunglobuline in oralen Leukoplakien und Karzinomen. *Dtsch. Z. Mund-Kiefer-Gesichts-Chir.* **1**, 168–177.

LŐRINCZY, E. (1956): The role of erythematous and catarrhal inflammations in developing leukoplakia. *Fogorv. Sz.* **49**, 182–185.

LŐRINCZY-LANDGRAF, E. (1947): Die erythematöse Entzündung der Mundschleimhaut. *Zschr. Stomat.* **44**, 1–11.

LŐRINCZY-LANDGRAF, E. (1958): Die erythematöse und katarrhalische Entzündung der Mundschleimhaut. *Dtsch. Zahnärztl. Z.* **13**, 921–929.

LUCY, J. A. and DINGLE, J. A. (1964): Fat soluble vitamins and biological membranes. *Nature* **204**, 156.

LUDY, J. B. and SHIRAZY, Z. E. (1941): Congenital leukokeratosis mucose oris. *Internat. Clin.* **4**, 38–41.

LUFT, J. H. (1961): Improvements in epoxy resin embedding methods. *J. Biophys. Biochem. Cytol.* **9**, 409–414.

LUZARDO-BAPTISTA, M. J. (1968): Leucoplasia del paladar. *Acta Odont. Venezulana* **6**, 5–19.

LUZARDO-BAPTISTA, M. J. and CASTEJON, O. J. (1968): Ultrastructura de las cellulas espinosas de la mucosa bucal humana normal. *Invest. Clin.* **27**, 17–38.

LUZARDO, M. J. and CASTEJON, O. J. (1969): Epithelial junction in the stratum spinosum of the human oral mucosa. *Parodontologia* **23**, 177–182.

LUZARDO-BAPTISTA, M. J. and GARCIA–TAMAYO, J. (1968): Ultrastructura de la lamina basal de las celules basales del epitelio de la mucosa bucal humana normal. *Invest. Clin.* **28**, 23–40.

LUZARDO-BAPTISTA, M. J. and GARCIA-TAMAYO, J. (1971*a*): Ultrastructura de la capa cornea en la mucosa bucal humana normal. *Invest. Clin.* **37**, 85–96.

LUZARDO-BAPTISTA, M. J, and GARCIA-TAMAYO, J. (1971*b*): Union intercellulares en mucosa humanes. *Invest. Clin.* **37**, 65–83.

LUZARDO-BAPTISTA, M. J. and GARCIA-TAMAYO, J. (1971*c*): Acid phosphatase activity in the small granules of epithelial cells in normal human oral mucosa. *Parodontologia* **25**, 49–55.

MACKENZIE, I. C. and MILES, A. E. M. (1973): The effect of chronic frictional stimulation on hamster cheek pouch epithelium. *Arch. Oral Biol.* **184**, 1341–1349.

MAIN, D. G. M. (1966): Mitotic activity in buccal keratoses. *Oral Surg.* **22**, 58–65.

MARSDEN, A. T. H. (1960): Betel cancer in Malaya. *Med. J. Malaysia* **14**, 162–168.

MARTIN, H. E. and HOWE, M. E. (1941): Glossitis rhombica mediana. *Ann. Surg.* **107**, 39–43.

MASKILLEJSON, A. (1969): Über die Vorkrebserkrankungen der Lippen. *Derm. Mschr.* **155**, 103–113.

MATHIS, H. (1964): Präkanzerosen der Mundschleimhäute. *Zahnärztl. Rdsch.* **73**, 321–330.

MATOLTSY, A. G. and PARAKKAL, P. P. (1965): Membrane-coating granules of keratinizing epithelia. *J. Cell Biol.* **24**, 297–307.

MATRAS, H. (1969): Zur Leukoplakie der Mundschleimhaut. *Zahnärztl. Welt/Rdsch.* **78**, 451–456.

MATSUMOTO, Y., UCHIDA, T., MARUYA, M., TOKITA, M., SETO, K. and WATANABE, Y. (1976): Scanning electron microscopic study of the human oral mucosa. *J. Dent. Res.* **55**, D. 176, 28.

MCCARTHY, F. (1941): A clinical and pathological study of oral diseases. *J. Am. Med. Ass.* **27**, 1950–1957.

MCCARTHY, P. L. and SHKLAR, G. (1964): *Diseases of the Oral Mucosa.* McGrew Hill, New York.

MCCLATCHEY, K. B., SILVERMAN, B. and HANSEN, L. (1975): Studies on oral lichen planus. *Oral. Surg.* **39**, 122–129.

MEHTA, F. S. and PINDBORG, J. J. (1974): Spontaneous remission of oral leukoplakias among Indian villagers in a 5-year follow-up study. *Community Dent. Oral Epidemiol.* **2**, 80–84.

MEHTA, F. S., DAFTARY, D. K. and SAHIAR, B. E. (1970): A correlative histocytological study of epithelial atypia in leukoplakia and submucous fibrosis lesions amongst Indian villagers in a mass screening programme. *Indian J. Cancer* **7**, 18.

MEHTA, F. S., PINDBORG, J. J. and HAMNER, J. E. (1971): *Oral Cancer and Precancerous Conditions in India,* Munksgaard, Copenhagen, p. 138.

MEHTA, F. S., DAFTARY, D. K., SHROFF, B. C. and SANGHVI, I. D. (1969*a*): Clinical and histological study of oral leukoplakia in relation to habits. A five-year follow-up. *Oral Surg.* **28**, 372–388.

MEHTA, F. S., PINDBORG, J. J., GUPTA, P. C. and DAFTARY, D. K. (1969*b*): Epidemiologic and histologic study of oral cancer and leukoplakia among 50,915 villagers in India. *Cancer* **24**, 832–849.

MEHTA, F. S., PINDBORG, J. J., DAFTARY, D. K. and GUPTA, P. C. (1969*c*): Oral leukoplakia among Indian villagers. The association with smoking habits. *Br. Dent. J.* **127**, 73–77.

MEHTA, F. S., SANJANA, M. K., SHROFF, B. C. and DOCTOR, R. H. C. (1961): Incidence of leukoplakia among "pan" (betel leaf) chewers and "bidi" smokers: a study of a sample survey. *Indian J. Med. Res.* **49**, 393–398.

MEHTA, F. S., SHROFF, B. C., GUPTA, P. C. and DAFTARY, D. K. (1972): Oral leukoplakia in relation to tobacco habits. A ten-year follow-up study of Bombay policemen. *Oral Surg.* **34**, 426–433.

MELA, F. L. (1965): La citologia esfoliativa nella diagnosi dei processi morbosi del cavo orale. *Minerva Stomatol.* **14**, 552–561.

MELA, F. and MONGINI, F. (1966*a*): Contributo casistico allo studio della leucoplachie orali. *Minerva Stomatol.* **15**, 502–507.

MELA, F. and MONGINI, F. (1966*b*): La terapia delle lesioni leucoplasiche del cavo orale (In base ai risultati di uno studio su 141 casi controllati a distanza dall'intervente). *Minerva Stomatol.* **15**, 804–811.

MELCZER, M. and KISS, GY. (1956): Data on development of leukoplakia oris. *Bőrgyógy. Vener. Sz.* **5**, 193–197.

MESKIN, L. H., REDMAN, R. S. and GORLIN, R. J. (1963): Incidence of geographic tongue among 3,668 students at the University of Minnesota. *J. Dent. Res.* **42**, 895–898.

MEYER, I. and SHKLAR, G. (1960): Multiple malignant tumours involving the oral mucosa and the gastrointestinal tract. *Oral Surg.* **13**, 295–299.

MEYER, J. (1967): Regional differences in human oral mucosa. *WHO Meeting of Investigators on Oral Precancerous Conditions, Copenhagen, 1967.*

MEYER, J., DAFTARY, D. K. and PINDBORG, J. J. (1967): Studies in oral leukoplakia. XI. Histopathology of leukoplakias in Indians chewing "pan" with tobacco. *Acta Odontol. Scand.* **25**, 397–435.

MEYER, J., MEDAK, H. and WEINMANN, J. P. (1960): Mitotic activity and rates of growth in regions of oral epithelium, differing in width. *Growth* **24**, 29–46.

MEYER, M. and SCHROEDER, H. E. (1975): A quantitative electron microscopic analysis of the keratinizing epithelium of normal human hard palate. *Cell Tiss. Res.* **158**, 177–189.

MIESCHER, G. (1943): Die Praecancerose der Haut und der angrenzenden Schleimhäute. *Schweiz, Med. Wschr.* **24**, 1072–1082.

MILLER, S. C., SOBERMAN, A. and STAHL, S. S. (1951): Study of the cornification of the oral epithelium by the use of oral scrapings. *J. Dent. Res.* **30**, 4–11.

MINCER, H. H., COLEMAN, S. A. and HOPKINS, K. P. (1972): Observations on the clinical characteristics of oral lesions showing histologic epithelial dysplasia. *Oral Surg.* **33**, 389–398.

MOERTEL, CH. G. and FOSS, E. L. (1958): Multicentric carcinomas of the oral cavity. *Surg. Gynec. Obstet.* **106**, 652–653.

MOERTEL, CH. G., DOCKERTY, M. B. and BAGGENSTOSS, A. H. (1961): Multiple primary malignant neoplasms. III. Tumours of multicentric origins. *Cancer*, **14**, 238.

MONTGOMERY, P. W. (1951): A study of exfoliative cytology of normal human oral mucosa. *J. Dent. Res.* **30**, 12–16.

MONTGOMERY, P. and HAAM, E. VON (1951): A study of the exfoliative cytology of oral leukoplakia. *J. Dent. Res.* **30**. 260–264.

MORGENROTH, K. (1963): Die Bewertung der Leukoplakien im Rahmen der Früherkennung bösartiger Veränderungen der Mundschleimhaut. *Schlesw. Holst. Aerztebl.* **16**, 1–6.

MORGENROTH, K. (1964): Precancerous changes in the oral cavity. *Acta Unio Internat. Cancer* **20**, 713–715.

MORGENROTH, K. and MORGENROTH, K. JR. (1970*a*): Untersuchungen von Mundschleimhautveränderungen mit dem Rasterelelektronenmikroskop. *Acta Mediotechn.* **18**, 18–23.

MORGENROTH, K. and MORGENROTH, K. JR. (1970*b*): Vergleichende stomatoskopische und rasterelektronenmikroskopische Untersuchungen von Mundschleimhautveränderungen. *Dtsch. Zahnärztl. Z.* **25**, 199–207.

MORGENROTH, K. and MORGENROTH, K. JR. (1970*c*): Rasterelektronenmikroskopische Untersuchungen zur Morphologie der Leukoplakie der Mundhöhle. *Dtsch. Zahnärztl. Z.* **25**, 1054–1060.

MORGENROTH, K. and THEMANN, H. (1962): Über den Glykogengehalt des Deckepithels der menschlichen Mundschleimhaut. *Dtsch Zahnärztl. Z.* **17**, 347–354.

MULAY, D. N. and URBACH, F. (1958;: Local therapy of oral leukoplakia with vitamin A. *Arch. Derm.* **78**, 637–641.

MUMFORD, O. B. and MORGAN, J. K. (1956): The use of cortison in lichen planus. *Br. J. Derm.* **68**, 258–260.

NATER, J. P., ZECCHA, J. J., HEIDA, F., PANDERS, A. K., CUYPERS, M., SAUER, E. W. and LINTUM, J. C. A. (1977): Floride orale Papillomatose, oder "speckled" Leukoplakie? *Der Hautarzt* **28**, 18–22.

NEUMANN-JENSEN, B., HOLMSTRUP, P. and PINDBORG, J. J. (1977): Smoking habits of 611 patients with oral lichen planus. *Oral Surg.* **43**, 410–415.

OBERMAYER, M. E. (1966): Cheek biting (Morsicatio buccarum). *Arch. Derm.* **90**, 185–190.

ODENS, M. (1967): Vitamin A and cancer. *Vitalstoff* **6**, 226–228.
ODLAND, G. P. (1960): A submicroscopic granular component in human epidermis. *J. Invest. Derm.* **34**, 11–15.
OHASHI, M., SAWADA, Y. and MAKITA, R. (1973): Odland body and intercellular substances. *Acta Derm. Venereol. Suppl. (Stockh.)* **73**, 47–54.
OHNSORGE, J. and HOLM, R. (1978): *Rasterelektronenmikroskopie*. Thieme, Stuttgart, p. 62.
ORBAN, B. and WENTZ, E. (1955): *Atlas of Clinical Pathology of Oral Mucous Membranes*. Mosby, St. Louis.
ORR, J. M. (1933): Oral cancer in betel nut chewers in Travancore. *Lancet* **11**, 575.
PALADE, G. E. (1952): A study of fixation for electron microscopy. *Exp. Med.* **95**, 285–298.
PAPANICOLAOU, G. and TRAUT, W. (1943): *Diagnosis of Uterine Cancer by the Vaginal Smear*. Commonwealth Fund, New York, pp. 5–7.
PAPE, H. D. (1970): Die Früherkennung der malignen Mundschleimhauttumoren unter besonderer Berücksichtigung der exfoliativen Zytologie. Habilitationschrift, Düsseldorf, Carl Hanser Verlag, München.
PASHKOV, B. H. and BELJAEVA, E.T. (1966): Soft leukoplakia in oral cavity. (in Russian) *Stomatologiia (Mosk.)* **45**, 3–6.
PAYNE, TH. F. (1975): Why are white lesions white? *Oral. Surg.* **40**, 652–658.
PETRZILKA, G. E. and SCHROEDER, H. E. (1976): Application of stereologic methodology to inflammatory infiltrates residing in oral mucous membrane lesions. *Beitr. Path. Bd.* **159**, 351–370.
PINDBORG, J. J. (1965): Oral cancer from an international point of view. *J. Can. Dent. Ass.* **31**, 219–226.
PINDBORG, J. J. (1968): *Atlas of Diseases of the Oral Mucosa*. Munksgaard, Copenhagen.
PINDBORG, J. J. (1971): Oral leukoplakia. *Aust. Dent. J.* **16**, 83–93.
PINDBORG, J. J. (1973): *Atlas of Diseases of the OralMucosa*. 2nd ed. Munksgaard, Copenhagen, pp. 56–57.
PINDBORG, J. J. (1977): Epidemiological studies of oral cancer. *Int. Dent. J.* **27**, 172–178.
PINDBORG, J. J. (1978): Oral cancer and precancer as diseases of the aged. *Community Dent. Oral Epidemol.* **6**, 300–307.
PINDBORG, J. J. (1980): *Oral Cancer and Precancer*. Wright J. Bristol, pp. 12–19.
PINDBORG, J. J. and RENSTRUP, G. (1963): Studies in oral leukoplakia. II. The effect of snuff on the oral epithelium. *Acta Derm. Venereol. (Stockh.)* **43**, 271–276.
PINDBORG, J. J. and ROED-PETERSEN, B. (1973): A follow-up study of 49 patients with epithelial dysplasia in oral leukoplakia. *WHO Meeting of Investigators of Oral Precancerous Conditions. Copenhagen, 1973.*
PINDBORG, J. J., BARMES, O. D. and ROED-PETERSEN, B. (1968): Epidemiology of leukoedema among Papuans and New-Guineans. *Cancer* **22**, 379–384.
PINDBORG, J. J., DAFTARY, D. K. and MEHTA, F. S. (1977): A follow-up study of sixty-one oral dysplastic precancerous lesions in Indian villagers. *Oral Surg.* **43**, 338–390.
PINDBORG, J. J., MEHTA, F. S. and DAFTARY, D. K. (1975): Incidence of oral cancer among 30,000 villagers in India in a 7-year follow-up study of oral precancerous lesions. *Community Dent. Oral Epidemiol.* **3**, 86–88.
PINDBORG, J. J., ROED-PETERSEN, B. and RENSTRUP, G. (1972): Role of smoking in floor of the mouth leukoplakias. *J. Oral Path.* **1**, 22–29.
PINDBORG, J. J., SHRIVASTAVA, A. N. and GUPTA, D. (1964): Studies in oral leukoplakias. VIII. Epithelial changes in tobacco induced leukoplakias in India. *Acta Odontol. Scand.* **22**, 499–512.

PINDBORG, J. J., JØLST, O., RENSTRUP, G. and ROED-PETERSEN, B. (1968): Studies in oral leukoplakia: a preliminary report on the period prevalence of malignant transformation in leukoplakia, based on a follow-up study of 248 patients. *J. Am. Dent. Ass.* **76**, 767–771.

PINDBORG, J. J., RENSTRUP, G., POULSEN, H. E. and SILVERMAN, S. (1963): Studies in oral leukoplakias: V. Clinical and histological signs of malignancy. *Acta Odontol. Scand.* **21**, 407–414.

PINDBORG, J. J., BHATT, M., DEVANATH, K. R., NARAYANA, H. R. and RAMACHANDRA, S. (1966): Frequency of oral white lesions among 10,000 individuals in Bangalore, South India. *Indian J. Med. Sci.* **20**, 349–352.

PINDBORG, J. J., CHAWLA, T. N., MISRA, R. K., NAGPAUL, R. K. and GUPTA, P. (1965*b*): Frequency of oral carcinoma, leukoplakia, leukokeratosis, leukoedema, submucous fibrosis and lichen planus in 10,000 Indians in Lucknow, Uttar Pradesh, India. *J. Dent. Res.* **44**, 615–618.

PINDBORG, J. J., KALAPESSI, H. K., KALE, S. A., SINGH, B. and TALVERKHAN, B. (1965*a*): Frequency of oral leukoplakias and related conditions among 10,000 Bombayites. *J. All India Dent. Ass.* **37**, 1–2.

PINDBORG, J. J., MEHTA, F. S., DAFTARY, D. K., GUPTA, P. C. and BHONSLEY, R. B. (1972): Prevalence of oral lichen planus among 7,639 Indian villagers in Kerala, South India. *Acta Derm.* **52**, 216–220.

PINDBORG, J. J., MEHTA, F. S., GUPTA, P. C., DAFTARY, D. K. and SMITH, C. J. (1971): Reverse smoking in Andhra Praedesh, India. A study of palatal lesions among 10,169 villagers. *Br. J. Cancer* **25**, 10–20.

PINKERT, R. (1967): Kritische Betrachtung zur Genese und Therapie der Glossitis rhombica mediana. *Dtsch. Stomatol.* **17**, 825–832.

PINKUS, H., JALLAD, M. and MELIREGAN, A. (1963): The inflammatory infiltrate of precancerous skin lesions. *J. Invest. Dermatol.* **41**, 247–255.

PLACKOVÁ, A., MEDAK, H., MEYER, J. and WATERHOUSE, J. P. (1971): Ultrastructure of surface cells of the oral mucosa. *Folia Morphol.* **19**, 165–170.

POLLIACK, A. and LEVIJ, I. S. (1969): The effect of topical vitamin A on papillomas and intraepithelial carcinoma induced in hamster cheek pouches with 9,10-Dimethyl-1, 2-benzanthracene. *Cancer Res.* **29**, 327–332.

POMERANZ, M. J. and STAHL, S. (1953): A correlative study of cytodiagnosis and biopsy. *Oral Surg.* **6**, 1026–1031.

POSWILLO, D. E. (1971): A comparative study of the effects of electrosurgery and cryosurgery in the management of benign oral lesions. *Br. J. Oral Surg.* **9**, 1–7.

PRINZ, H. (1928): Tobacco and leukoplakia oris. *Dent. Record* **48**, 521.

PRINZ, R. (1927): Wandering rash of the tongue. *Dent. Cosmos* **69**, 272–275.

RAHAMIMOFF, F. and MUHSAM, H. V. (1957): Some observations on 1,246 cases of geographic tongue. *Am. J. Dis. Child.* **93**, 519–525.

REDDY, C. R. R. M. and KAMESWARI, V. R. (1974): Oral exfoliative cytology in reverse smokers having carcinoma of hard palate. *Acta Cytol.* **18**, 201–204.

REDMAN R. S. (1970): Prevalence of geographic tongue, fissured tongue, median rhomboid glossitis and hairy tongue among the Minnesota school children. *Oral Surg.* **30**, 390–395.

REDMAN, R. S., VANCE, F. L., GORLIN, R. J., PENGLER, F. D. and MESKIN, L. H. (1966): Physiological component in the etiology of geographic tongue. *J. Dent. Res.* **45**, 1403 1408.

REHRMANN, A. and PAPE, H. D. (1966): Die operative Behandlung der Präkanzerosen. *Arch. Klin. Dermat.* **227**, 819–824.

RENNEFAHRT, I. and KUNZE, P. (1969): Beitrag zur Leukoplakie der Mundschleimhaut. *Dtsch. Stomatol.* **19**, 81–90.

RENSTRUP, G. (1958): Leukoplakia of the oral cavity. *Acta Odontol. Scand.* **16**, 99–111.

RENSTRUP, G. (1963): Studies in oral leukoplakias. IV. Mitotic activity in oral leukoplakias. *Acta Odontol. Scand.* **21**, 333–340.

RENSTRUP, G. (1970): Occurrence of Candida in oral leukoplakias. *Acta Pathol. Microbiol. Scand. (B)* **78**, 421–424.

RENSTRUP, G. and PINDBORG, J. J. (1958): Oral manifestation in lichen ruber planus *Ugeskr. Laeger.* **120**, 1327–1330.

REYNOLDS, E. S. (1963): The use of lead citrate at high pH as an electron-opaque stain in electron microscopy. *J. Cell Biol.* **17**, 208–213.

RHEINWALD, U. (1956): Bioelektrische Metallwirkungen in der Mundhöhle. *Z. Stomatol.* **53**, 519–526.

RHEINWALD, W., MAYER, H., THIELEMANN, K. and LOEBICH, O. (1954): Die Wahrheit über das Problem der galvanischen Elemente im Mund. *Zahnärztl. Mitt.* No. **24**/54.

RHODIN, J. (1954): *Correlation of ultrastructural organization and function in normal and experimentally changed proximal convoluted tubule cells of the mouse kidney.* Thesis, AB Goodwill, Stockholm.

RICHARDSON, E. R. (1968): Incidence of geographic tongue and median rhomboid glossitis in 3,319 Negro college students. *Oral Surg.* **26**, 623–625.

RITZAU, M. (1971): Naevus spongiosus albus mucosae. *Tandlaegebladet* **75**, 690–709.

ROED-PETERSEN, B. (1971): Cancer development in oral leukoplakia. Follow-up of 331 patients. *J. Dent. Res.* **50**, 711–716.

ROED-PETERSEN, B. and PINDBORG, J. J. (1973): A study of Danish snuff-induced oral leukoplakias. *J. Oral Path.* **2**, 301–313.

ROED-PETERSEN, B. and RENSTRUP, G. (1969): A topographical classification of the oral mucosa suitable for electronic data processing (its application to 560 leukoplakias). *Acta Odontol. Scand.* **27**, 681–695.

ROED-PETERSEN, B., BÁNÓCZY, J. and PINDBORG, J. J. (1973): Smoking habits and histological characteristics of oral leukoplakias in Denmark and Hungary. *Br. J. Cancer* **28**, 575–579.

ROED-PETERSEN, B., GUPTA, P. C., PINDBORG, J. J. and SINGH, B. (1972): Association between oral leukoplakia and sex, age and tobacco habits. *Bull. WHO* **47**, 13–19.

ROED-PETERSEN, B., RENSTRUP, G. and PINDBORG, J. J. (1970): Candida in oral leukoplakia. *Scand. J. Dent. Res.* **78**, 323–328.

ROED-PETERSEN, B., ROED-PETERSEN, J. and BENDIXEN, G. (1973): Cell mediate immunity to human oral leukoplakia demonstrated by the leukocyte migration test. *Int. J. Cancer* **12**. 66–72.

ROSENTHAL, W. (1962): Die fakultativen Präkanzerosen. *Dtsch. Stomatol.* **12**, 653–663.

RUBINSTEIN, A. B., MEDAK, H. and MEYER, J. (1970): Early effects of smoking on surface cytology of the oral mucosa. *Oral Surg.* **30**, 131–141.

RUBIO, C. A. and KRANTZ, I. (1976): The exfoliating cervical epithelial surface in dysplasia, carcinoma in situ and invasive squamous carcinoma. I. Scanning electron microscopic study. *Acta Cytol.* **20**, 144–150.

RUDELT, H. G. and PETERS, K. R. (1978): Vergleichende Licht- und Rasterelektronenmikroskopische Untersuchungen der menschlichen Gingiva mit der Filter–Imprint Methode. *Dtsch. Zahnärztl. Z.* **33**, 375–383.

SALIS-SAMADEN, R. (1965): Beitrag zur Strahlentherapie der oralen Leukoplakie. *Strahlentherapie* **125**, 426–430.

SALLAY, K. (1969): Treatment of lichen oris with hydrocortison-microcrystal suspension given intrafocally. *Fogorv. Sz.* **62,** 257–260.

SALLAY, K. and CSIBA, Á. (1973): Tongue carcinoma. Two rare cases. *Fogorv. Sz.* **66,** 199–204.

SAMMAN, P. D. (1956): A note on the natural history of lichen planus. *Br. J. Derm.* **68,** 175–181.

SAMMET, J. F. (1940): Median rhomboid glossitis. *Radiology,* **32,** 215. 1939. *cit.* by *Zbl. Nas-Ohrenheilk.,* **33,** 61, 1940.

SANDLER, H. C., STAHL, S S.,. CAHN, L. R. and FREUND, H. R. (1960): Exfoliative cytology for detection of early mouth cancer. *Oral Surg.* **13,** 994–1009.

SANDSTEAD, H. R. and LOWE, J. W. (1953): Leukoedema and keratosis in relation to leukoplakia of the buccal mucosa in man. *J. Nat. Cancer Inst.* **14,** 423–437.

SATO, A. and SEIJI, M. (1973): Electron microscopic observation of malignant dyskeratosis in leukoplakia and Bowen's disease. *Acta Derm. Venereol. (Suppl.) (Stockh.)* **73,** 101–110.

SCHAFF, ZS., LAPIS, K. and BEREZESKY, I. K. (1974): The scanning electron microscopy as a new testing method; its role and application in medical science. *Orv. Hetil.* **22,** 1263–1267.

SCHENK, P. (1975): *Die ultrastrukturelle Morphologie normalen und pathologischen oralen Epithelien unter besonderer Berücksichtigung von dysplastischen und dyskeratotischen Veränderungen, Carcinoma in situ und invasivem Carcinom.* Thesis, Stockholm.

SCHENK, P. and WERSÄLL, J. (1975): Ultrastruktur der Papillae filiformes der menschlichen Zunge. *Arch. Derm. Forsch.* **252,** 91–109.

SCHETTLER, D. and KOBERG, W. (1970): Zur malignen Entartung des Lichen ruber planus der Mundschleimhaut. *Dtsch. Zahnärztl. Z.* **25,** 991–992.

SCHMIDT, H. (1961): Frequency, duration and localisation of lichen planus. *Acta Derm. Venereol. (Stockh.)* **41,** 181–187.

SCHRIEVER, W. and DIAMOND, L. (1952): Electromotive forces and electric currents caused by metallic dental fillings. *J. Dent. Res.* **31,** 205–229.

SCHROEDER, H. E. (1973): Transmigration and infiltration of leukocytes in human junctional epithelium. *Helv. Odontol. Acta* **17,** 6–18.

SCHROEDER, H. E. and MÜNZEL-PEDRAZZOLI, S. (1970): Morphometric analysis comparing junctional and oral epithelium of normal human gingiva. *Helv. Odontol. Acta* **14,** 53–66.

SCHROEDER, H. E. and MÜNZEL-PEDRAZZOLI, S. (1973): Correlated morphometric and biochemical analysis of gingival tissue. *J. Microscopy* **99,** 301–329.

SCHROEDER, H. E., KLEIN-SZÁNTÓ, A. J. P. and BÁNÓCZY, J. (1978): Leukoplakia simplex, oder metaplastische Keratose der Mundschleimheut? *Zahn, Mund Kieferheilk.* **66,** 141–154.

SCHUERMANN, H. (1958): *Krankheiten der Mundschleimhaut und der Lippen.* Urban u. Schwarzenberg, München–Berlin, pp. 277–279.

SCHUERMANN, H., GREITHER, A. and HORNSTEIN, O. (1966): *Krankheiten der Mundschleimhaut und der Lippen.* Urban u. Schwarzenberg, München–Berlin–Wien, p. 42.

SCHWENZER, N. (1968): Konservative und operative Behandlung der Leukoplakie der Mundhöhle. *Fortschr. Kiefer. Gesichtschir.* Vol. XIII. pp. 140–145.

SCHWIMMER, E. (1877): Some rare clinical pictures of oral and lingual mucosa. *Orv. Egyesület Évkönyve, 1877, Nr. 48.*

SCOTT, C. R. (1966): Hereditary leukokeratosis, white mouth. *J. Pediatr.* **68,** 768–772.

SEIFERT, G. and BURKHARDT, A. (1979): Orale Krebsvorstadien. *Verh. Dtsch. Ges. Path.* **63,** 74–96.

Seifert, G. and Vossmeyer, M. (1978): Glossitis rhombica mediana. (Brocq) Pathologisch-anatomische Analyse von 28 Fällen. *Dtsch. Z. Mund-Kiefer-Gesichts-Chir.* **2,** 162–170.

Sewerin, I. E. (1971): A clinical and epidemiologic study of morsicatio buccarum/labiorum. *Scand. J. Dent. Res.* **79.** 73–80.

Shafer, W. G. (1967): The use of the term "Leukoplakia". *Meeting Invest. Oral Precanc. Cond. 7–12. Aug. 1967, Copenhagen.*

Shafer, W. G. (1975): Oral carcinoma in situ. *Oral Surg.* **39,** 227–238.

Shafer, W. G. (1980): Basic clinical features of oral premalignant lesions. In: *Oral Premalignancy.* Ed by J. C. Mackenzie, E. Dabelsteen and Ch. A. Squier. University of Iowa Press, Iowa City, pp. 15–22.

Shafer, W. G. and Standish, S. M. (1965): Oral exfoliative cytology. *J. Indiana State Dent. Assoc.* **44,** 143.

Shafer, W. G. and Waldron, Ch. A. (1961): A clinical and histopathological study of oral leukoplakia. *Surg. Gynecol. Obstet.* **112,** 411–420.

Shafer, W. G., Hine, M. K. and Levy, B. M. (1974): *A Textbook of Oral Pathology.* Saunders, Philadelphia, p. 94.

Sharp, G. S. (1956): Abnormal mucous membranes, as related to oral cancer. *Cancer Unio Internat. contra Cancrum,* **12,** 135–139.

Sharp, G. S. and Bullock, W. K. (1958): Carcinoma arising in glossitis rhombica mediana. *Cancer* **11,** 149–149.

Sharp, G. S., Bullock, W. K. and Helsper, G. W. (1961): Multiple oral carcinoma. *Cancer* **14,** 512–514.

Shillitoe, E. I., Greenspan, J. S. and Silverman, S. (1980): Herpes simplex virus antibodies in leukoplakia and oral cancer. *J. Dent. Res.* **59,** 332.

Shillitoe, E. J. and Silverman, S. (1979): Oral cancer and herpes simplex virus — a review. *Oral Surg.* **48,** 216–224.

Shklar, G. (1972): Lichen planus as an oral ulcerative disease. *Oral Surg.* **33,** 376–388.

Shklar, G. and McCarthy, Ph. (1961): The oral lesions of lichen planus. *Oral Surg.* **14,** 164–174.

Shklar, G. and Meyer, J. (1961): The histopathology and histochemistry of dermatological lesions in the mouth. *Oral Surg.* **14,** 1069–1084.

Shklar, G., Meyer, J., Cataldo, E. and Taylor, R. (1968): Correlated study of oral cytology and histopathology. *Oral Surg.* **25,** 61–71.

Silverman, J. (1967): Ultrastructure studies of oral mucosa. I. Comparison of normal and hyperkeratotic human buccal epithelium. *J. Dent. Res.* **46,** 1433–1443.

Silverman, S. (1959): Detection of intraoral carcinoma in situ with exfoliative cytology. *J. Dent. Res.* **38,** 717.

Silverman, S. and Galante, M. (1972): *Oral Cancer.* University of California, San Francisco, pp. 8–13.

Silverman, S. and Griffith, M. (1972): Smoking characteristics of patients with oral carcinoma and the risk for second oral primary carcinoma. *J. Am. Dent. Assoc.* **85,** 637–640.

Silverman, S. and Griffith, M. (1974): Studies on lichen planus. *Oral Surg.* **37,** 705–710.

Silverman, S. and Rozen, R. D. (1968): Observations on the clinical characteristics and natural history of oral leukoplakia. *J. Am. Dent. Assoc.* **76,** 772–776.

Silverman, S. and Ware, W. H. (1960): Comparison of histologic, cytologic and clinical findings in intraoral leukoplakia and associated carcinoma. *Oral Surg.* **13,** 412–422.

SILVERMAN, S., BARBOSA, J. and KEARNS, G. (1971): Ultrastructural and histochemical localisation of glycogen in human normal and hyperkeratotic oral epithelium. *Arch. Oral Biol.* **16**, 423–434.
SILVERMAN, S., BECKS, H. and FARBER, S. M. (1958): The diagnostic value of intraoral cytology. *J. Dent. Res.* **37**, 195–205.
SILVERMAN, S., RENSTRUP, G. and PINDBORG, J. J. (1963a)! Studies in oral leukoplakias. III. Effects of vitamin A comparing clinical, histopathological, cytologic and hematologic responses. *Acta Odontol. Scand.* **21**, 271–292.
SILVERMAN, S., RENSTRUP, G. and PINDBORG, J. J. (1963b): Studies in oral leukoplakias. VII. Further investigations on the effects of vitamin A on keratinization. *Acta Odontol. Scand.* **21**, 553–570.
SILVERMAN, S., BHARGAVA, K., MANI, N., SMITH, L. W. and MALAOWALLA, A. M. (1976): Malignant transformation and natural history of oral leukoplakia in 57,518 industrial workers of Gujarat, India. *Cancer* **38**, 1790–1795.
SILVERMAN, S., BILIMORIA, K. F., BHARGAVA, K., MANI, N. J. and SHAH, R. (1977): Cytologic, histologic and clinical correlations of precancerous and cancerous oral lesions in 57,518 industrial workers of Gujarat, India. *Acta Cytol.* **21**, 196–198.
SIMPSON, H. E. (1957): The age and sex incidence and anatomical distribution of oral leukoplakia and lichen planus. *Br. J. Derm.* **69**, 178–180.
SIMSA, J. (1955): Mereni elektryckych proudu na kovoych nahredach v ustech. *Csl. Stomatol.* **1**, 13–15.
SKACH, M., SVOBODA, O. and KUBÁT, K. (1960): Prisperich k problému leukoplakie. *Acta Univ. Carol. Sect. Med. Suppl.* **10**, 363–371.
SMITH, C. J. and RENSTRUP, G. (1970): The chronic inflammatory cell reactions associated with oral leukoplakia. *Meeting Invest. Oral Precanc. Cond.* 19–33. *Jan. 1970, Bombay.*
SMITH, J. F. (1962a): Clinical evaluation of massive buccal vitamin A dosage in oral hyperkeratosis. *Oral Surg.* **15**, 282–292.
SMITH, J. F. (1962b): White sponge nevus report of case. *J. Oral. Surg.* **20**, 153–155.
SMITH, J. F., MINCER, H. A., HOPKINS, K. P. and BELL, J. (1970): Snuffdipper's lesion. A clinical and pathological study in a large population. *Arch. Otolaryngol.* **92**, 450–456.
SOGNNAES, R. F. and ALBRIGHT, J. T. (1956): Preliminary observations on the fine structure of oral mucosa. *Anat. Rec.* **126**, 225–232.
SOGNNAES, R. F. and ALBRIGHT, J. T. (1958): Electron microscopy of the epithelial lining of the human oral mucosa. *Oral Surg.* **11**, 662–673.
SOLOMON, H. A. and REINHARD, M. C. (1943): Electrical currents from dental metals as etiological factors in oral cancer. *Am. J. Cancer* **22**, 606–609.
SONKODI, I. (1976): Cryotherapy in stomato-oncology. *Magy. Onkol.* **20**, 48–52.
SONKODI, I. and BÁNÓCZY, J. (1976): Morsicatio buccarum et labiorum. *Fogorv. Sz.* **67**, 165–169.
SONKODI, I. and BODA, K. (1977): Data on morbity of oral precarcinomas, with special regard to white lesions. *Fogorv. Sz.* **70**, 257–262.
SONKODI, I. and GYŐRI, I. (1975): Histological evaluation of data of keratosis and lichen planus cases by the aid of computer analysis. *Fogorv. Sz.* **68**, 215–219.
SONKODI, I. and KESZTHELYI, G. (1975): Cryosurgery in stomatology. *Fogorv. Sz.* **68**, 234–237.
SONKODI, I. and TÓTH, K. (1973): Stomato-oncological examination of textile workers in Szeged. *Fogorv. Sz.* **66**, 506–509.

SPIESSL, B. and METZ, H. J. (1967): Differentialdiagnose und Behandlung der Leukoplakie. *Zahn, Mund Kieferheilk.* **48,** 1/2, 11–20.

SPRAGUE, W. G. (1963): A survey of the use of the term "leukoplakia" by oral pathologists. *Oral Surg.* **16,** 1067–1074.

SQUIER, C. A. (1970): Lysosomes in oral epithelium: the ultrastructural localisation of acid phosphatase and nonspecific esterase in keratinized oral epithelium in man and rat. *Arch. Oral Biol.* **15,** 153–168.

Statisztikai Évkönyv **1960**. Statisztikai Kiadó, Budapest 1961, p. 538.

Statisztikai Évkönyv **1970**. Statisztikai Kiadó, Budapest 1971, p. 573.

STRASSBURG, M. and KNOLLE, G. (1968): *Farbatlas der Mundschleimhauterkrankungen.* Quintessenz, Berlin, p. 18.

SUGÁR, J. (1961): Pathological nomenclature of dermal precancerosis. *Magy. Onkol.* **5,** 178–181.

SUGÁR, J. (1968): *Cell alterations during carcinogenesis and in tumours damaged by chemotherapy.* Thesis, Budapest, pp. 92–146.

SUGÁR, J. and FARAGÓ, L. (1967): Electron microscopic examination on morphogenesis of laryngeal carcinoma. *Morph. Igazságügyi Sz.* **7,** 81–89.

SUGÁR, L. (1959): *Oral Diseases.* Medicina, Budapest, pp. 223–225.

SUGÁR, L. and BÁNÓCZY, J. (1957): Investigations on precancerosis of oral mucosa. *Fogorv. Sz.* **50,** 347–353.

SUGÁR, L. and BÁNÓCZY, J. (1959): Untersuchungen bei Präkanzerose der Mundschleimhaut. *Zahn, Mund, Kieferheilk.* **30,** 132–140.

SUGÁR, L. and BÁNÓCZY, J. (1969): Follow-up studies in oral leukoplakia. *Bull. WHO* **41,** 289–293.

SUGÁR, L. and BÁNÓCZY, J. (1970*a*): Relationship between leukoplakia and carcinoma. *Fogorv. Sz.* **63,** 225–231.

SUGÁR, L. and BÁNÓCZY, J. (1970*b*): Leucoplasie et cancer. *Méd. Hyg.* **28,** 1468–1470.

SUGÁR, L. and BÁNÓCZY, J. (1970*c*): Observatii asupra unei boli a mucosaei bucal: Leucoedema exfoliativum mucosae oris. *Stomatologia (Bucureşti)* **17,** 199–204.

SUGÁR, L. and BÁNÓCZY, J. (1971): Leukoedema exfoliativum mucosae oris. *Fogorv. Sz.* **64,** 377–379.

SUGÁR, L. and BÁNÓCZY, J. (1975): Change in clinical types of oral leukoplakia. *Fogorv. Sz.* **68,** 257–260.

SUGÁR, L., BÁNÓCZY, J., RÁCZ, I. and SALLAY, K. (1975): *Oral Diseases.* Medicina, Budapest, pp. 157–170.

SVEJDA, J. and JANOTA, M. (1974): Scanning electron microscopy of the papillae foliate of the human tongue. *Oral Surg.* **37,** 208–216.

SVEJDA, J., SKACH, M. and PLACKOVÁ, A. (1977): Hairlike variations of filiform papillae in the human tongue. *Oral Surg.* **43,** 97–105.

SYMEONIDIS, A. (1969): Leukoplakia from the histopathologic viewpoint and its relation to oral carcinoma. *Stomatologia (Athen)* **26,** 5–12.

SZODORAY, L. (1963): Cheilitis caused by light, as precancerosis. *Magy. Onkol.* **7,** 20–24.

SZODORAY, L. and SZABÓ, P. (1972): Experiences in field of radiotherapy concerning dermal basaliomas. *Orvosképzés* **47,** 239–244.

TAKENAGA, A., MATSUDA, M., HORAI, T., IKEGANNI, H. and HATTORI, SH. (1977): Scanning electron microsopy in the study of lung cancer. *Acta Cytol.* **21,** 90–95.

TARNAI, K. and ZÁRAY, E. (1953*a*): Das Verhalten der Metalle im Organismus. *Zahn, Mund, Kieferheilk.* **18,** 215–220.

TARNAI, K. and ZÁRAY, E. (1953*b*): Behaviour of metals in the organism. *Fogorv. Sz.* **46,** 48–53.

TEMPEL, V. (1972): Beitrag zur Frage der malignen Entartung von Leukoplakien der Mundhöhle. *Dtsch. Stomatol.* **22**, 814–820.

TENTSCHOV, G. and ANDREJEW, V. I. (1956): Behandlung der Leukoplakie der Mundhöhle durch Nahbestrahlung. *Strahlentherapie* **99**, 364–368.

THEMANN, H. (1958): Elektronenmikroskopische Untersuchungen der normalen und pathologisch veränderten Mundschleimhaut. *Fortschr. Kiefer Gesichtschir.* **4**, 390–394.

THOMA, K. and GOLDMAN, H. (1960): *Oral Pathology.* Mosby, St. Louis, pp. 1443–1460.

TIECKE, R. W. and BERNIER, J. L. (1954): Statistical and morphological analysis of four hundred and one cases of intraoral squamous cell carcinoma. *J. Am. Dent. Assoc.* **49**, 684–698.

TIECKE, R. W. and BLOZIS, G. G. (1966): Oral cytology. *J. Am. Dent. Assoc.* **72**, 855–861.

TOURAINE, A. and BAUDOUIN, A. G. (1937): Trois observations de leucoplasie electrogalvanique, dont une avec cancer. *Bull. Soc. Franc. Dermatol. Syph.* **44**, 2066.

TROTT, J. R. and BÁNÓCZY, J. (1962): The oral mucosa and keratinization. *Acta Morph. Hung.* **11**, 217–228.

TURESKY, S., GLICKMAN, L. and PROVOST, J. (1961): A histochemical study of the keratotic process in oral lesions diagnosed clinically as leukoplakia. *Oral. Surg.* **14**, 442–453.

TURPIN, H. and CARATZALI, A. (1936): Contribution à l'étiologie de la glossite exfoliatrice marginée. *Presse Méd.* **64**, 1273–1274.

ULLMANN, K. (1932): Über seltene und neue Formen der Leukoplakia mucosae oris. *Wien Klin. Wschr.* **45**, 840–852.

UMIKER, W. O., LAMPE, I., RAPP, R. and HINIKER, J. (1960): Oral smears in the diagnosis of carcinoma and premalignant lesions. *Oral Surg.* **13**, 897–907.

UNNA, P. G. (1881): Über kreisfleckige Exfoliation der Hohlhand und der Zunge. *Arch. Derm.* **13**, 295–302.

VAKILZADEK, F. (1967): Zur Morsicatio labiorum. *Z. Hautkr.* **42**, 253–256.

VAN DER WAAL, I., BEEMSTER, G. and VAN DER KWAST, W. A. M. (1979): Median rhomboid glossitis caused by Candida? *Oral Surg.* **47**, 31–35.

VÁNDOR, F. (1969): *Diagnosis and Therapy of Tumours of the Oral Cavity, Pharynx and Upper Respiratory System.* Thesis, Budapest.

VÁNDOR, F. (1978): *Tumours of the Oral Cavity.* Medicina, Budapest pp. 113, 121.

VENKEI, T. and SUGÁR, J. (1965): *Early Diagnosis, Pathohistology and Treatment of Malignant Tumours of the Skin.* Akadémiai Kiadó, Budapest pp. 39–45.

WAECHTER, R. (1978): Technik und Indikation der Zytodiagnostik für die Früherkennung des Karzinoms. *Schweiz, Mschr. Zahnheilk.* **88**, 829–836.

WAHI, P. N. and MITAL, V. P. (1970): Epidemiological study of precancerous lesions of the oral cavity: a preliminary report. *Indian J. Med. Res.* **58**, 1361–1391.

WAHI, P. N., PATH, F. C., KEHAR, USHA and PATH, M. C. (1966): Morphological and cytochemical studies of cells of precancerous lesions of the oral cavity. *Acta Cytol.* **10**, 173.

WALDRON, CH. A. (1965): Oral leukoplakia, carcinoma and the prosthodontist. *J. Prosthet. Dent.* **15**. 367–376.

WALDRON, CH. A. and SHAFER, W. G. (1960): Current concepts of leukoplakia. *Int. Dent. J.* **10**. 350–367.

WALDRON, CH. A. and SHAFER, W. G. (1975): Leukoplakia revisited. A clinicopathologic study of 3,256 oral leukoplakias. *Cancer* **36**, 1386–1392.

WANNENMACHER, M. F., TETSCH, P. and ESSER, E. (1972): Behandlung der Leukoplakie mit subtoxischen Vitamin-A-Dosen. *Dtsch. Zahnärztl. Z.* **27**, 154–158.

WARD, G. E. (1953): Leukoplakia. *Bull. Canc. Prog. Am. Canc. Soc.* **3**, 131.
WARIN, R. P., CRABB, H. S. M. and DARLING, A. J. (1958): Lichen planus of the mouth. *Br. Med. J.* **1**, 938–948.
WATSON, M. L. (1958): Staining of tissue sections for electron microscopy with heavy metals. *J. Biophys. Biochem. Cytol.* **4**, 475–478.
WEIBEL, E. R. (1969): Stereologic principles for morphometry in electron microscopic cytology. *Int. Rev. Cytol.* **26**, 235–246.
WEIBEL, E. R. (1970): An automatic sampling stage microscope for stereology. *J. Microscopy.* **91**, 1–12.
WEIBEL, E. R. and BOLENDER, R. P. (1973): Stereological Techniques for Electron Microscopic Morphometry. In: *Principles and Techniques of Electron Microscopy.* Vol. 3. Ed. by M. E. Hayat. Van Nostrand Rheinhold Comp., New York, p. 237.
WEIBEL, E. R., KISTLER, G. S. and SCHERLE, V. P. (1966): Practical stereologic methods on morphometric cytology. *J. Cell. Biol.* **30**, 23–34.
WEINER, A. L. (1969): White sponge nevus: familial-congenital leukokeratosis mucosae oris. *Cutis* **5**, 555–558.
WEINMANN, J. P. (1940): Keratinization of the human oral mucosa. *J. Dent. Res.* **19**, 57–72.
WEISBERGER, D. (1957): Precancerous lesions. *J. Am. Dent. Assoc.* **54**, 507–508.
WEISMAN, G. (1965): Lysosomes. *New England J. Med.* **273**, 1084–1090.
WELSH, A. L. (1955): *Differential Diagnosis of Leukoplakia, Leukokeratosis and Cancer in the Mouth.* Thomas, Springfield, p. 62.
WHITTAKER, D. K. and ADAMS, D. (1971): The surface layer of human foetal skin and oral mucosa: a study by scanning and transmission electron microscopy. *J. Anat.* **108**, 453–464.
WHITTEN, J. B. (1970): The electron microscopic examination of congenital keratoses of the oral mucous membrane. *Oral Surg.* **29**, 69–84.
W.H.O. Collaborating Centre for Oral Precancerous Lesions: (1978): Definition of leukoplakia and related lesions: An aid to studies on oral precancer. *Oral Surg.* **46**, 518–539.
WILL, W. (1966): *Naeviforme isolierte hypertropische Mundschleimhautkeratosen.* Inaug. Diss. Köln.
WILSCH, L., HORNSTEIN, O. P., BRÜNING, H., SCHWIPPER, V., LÖSEL, F., SCHÖNBERGER, A., GUNSELMANN, W. and PRESTELE, H. (1978): Orale Leukoplakien. II. Ergebnisse einer 1-jährigen poliklinischen Pilotstudie. *Dtsch. Zahnärztl. Z.* **33**, 132–142.
WINIKER-BLANCK, E. (1961): Die Leukoplakia oris als Präkanzerose. *Dtsch. Stomatol.* **11**, 368–373.
WITKOP, C. J. and GORLIN, R. J. (1961): Four hereditary mucosal syndromes. Comparative histology and exfoliative cytology of Darier–White's disease, hereditary benign intraepithelial dyskeratosis, white sponge nevus and pachyonychia. *Arch. Derm. Syph.* **84**, 762–771.
WOLFF, K. and HOLUBAR, K. (1968): Odland Körper als epidermale Lysosomen: ein elektronen-mikroskopisch cytochemischer Beitrag zum Verhornungsprozess der Haut. *Arch. Klin. Exp. Derm.* **231**, 1–9.
WORLD HEALTH ORGANIZATION (1980): *Oral Mucosa Manual.* Geneva.
WRUBEL, G. J. and SCOPP, W. (1961): A study of the exfoliative cytology of the hard palate and buccal mucosa following cessation of smoking in previous smokers. *J. Dent. Res.* **40**, 341–345.
ZACHARIAH, J., MATTHEW, B., VARMA, N. A. R., IZBAL, A. M. and PINDBORG, J. J.

(1966): Frequency of oral mucosal lesions among 5,000 individuals in Trivandrum, South India. *J. All India Dent. Assoc.* **38**, 290–294.

ZEGARELLI, E. V. and KUTSCHER, A. H. (1957): Familial white folded hypertrophy of the mucous membranes. Report of three cases. *Oral Surg.* **10**, 262–270.

ZEGARELLI, E. V., KUTSCHER, A. H. and HYMAN, G. A. (1969): *Diagnoses of Diseases of the Mouth and Jaws.* Lea and Febiger, Philadelphia, pp. 461–463.

ZEGARELLI, E. V., EVERETT, F. G., KUTSCHER, A. H., GORMAN, A. H. and KUPFERBERG, N. (1959): Familial white folded dysplasia of the mucous membranes. *Arch. Derm. Syph. (Chicago)* **80**, 97–103.

ZEGARELLI, E. V., KUTSCHER, A. R., MERCADENTE, J. A., NAPOLI, N. and IURNO, E. (1963): Geographic tongue, relation of changes in appearance to time. *Dent. Abstr.* **8**, 421–431.

ZELICKSON, A. S. (1961): Normal human keratinization processes as demonstrated by electron microscopy. *J. Invest. Dermatol.* **37**, 369–379.

ZELICKSON, A. S. and HARTMANN, J. F. (1962): An electron microscopy study of normal human nonkeratinizing oral mucosa. *J. Invest. Derm.* **38**, 99–103.

ZIMMERMANN, E. and ZIMMERMANN, A. (1965): Effect of race, age, smoking habits and oral systemic disease on oral exfoliative cytology. *J. Dent. Res.* **44**, 627–631.

COLOUR PHOTOS

Colour photo 1. Simple leukoplakia with a pavement-like pattern of hyperkeratosis on the dorsum of the tongue of a 62-year-old male patient

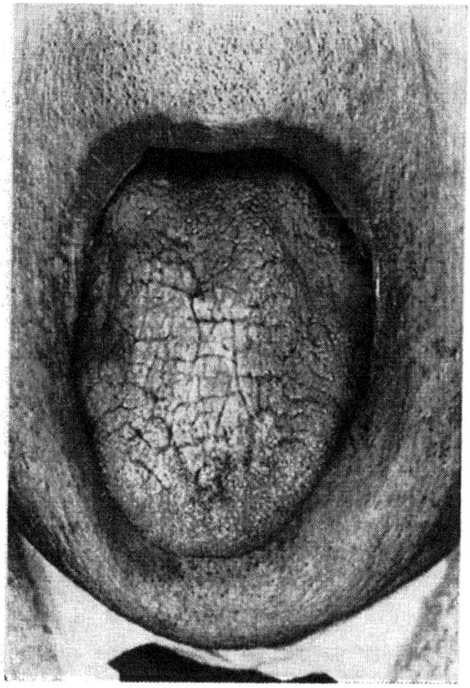

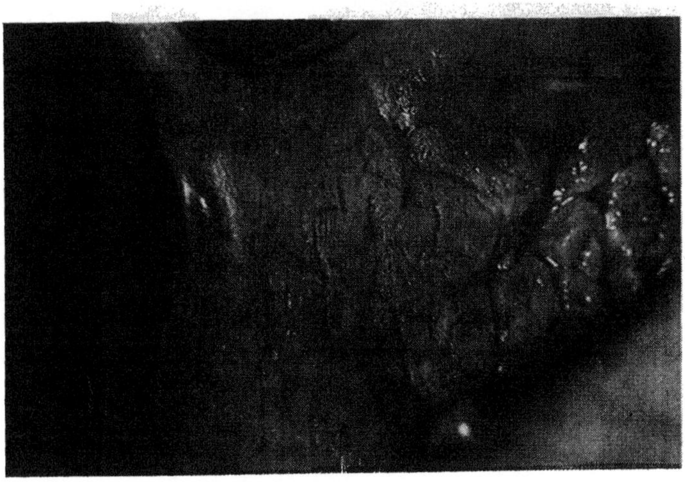

Colour photo 2. Simple leukoplakia in the buccal mucosa of an 50-year-old male patient. The changed area shows a mosaic-like hyperkeratosis and is slightly elevated

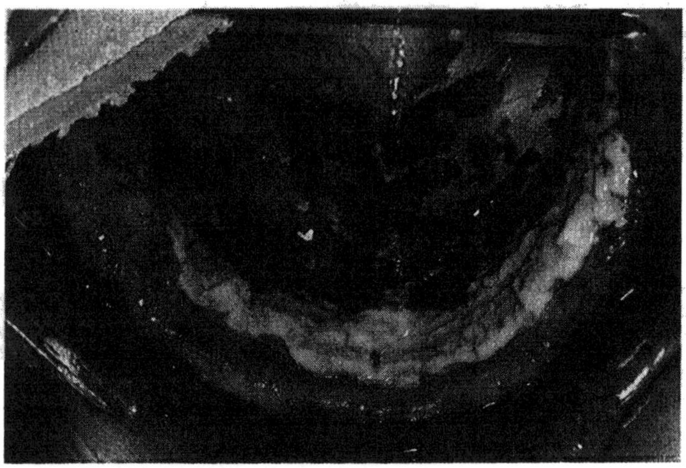

Colour photo 3. Extensive verrucous leukoplakia on the floor of the mouth and on the lingual part of the alveolar ridge of a 77-year-old male patient who had been a heavy smoker but who did not wear prosthesis

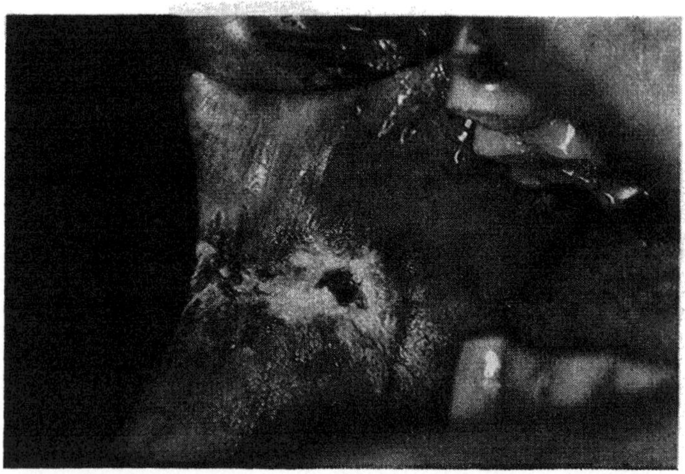

Colour photo 4. Erosive leukoplakia due to mechanical irritation and candidiasis in the oral commissure of a 43-year-old male patient

Colour photo 5. Migratory glossitis in a 20-year-old female patient. Hyperaemic spots are located on the tip and margins of the tongue, but had changed their position several times. The filiform papillae are destroyed but the fungiform papillae are preserved

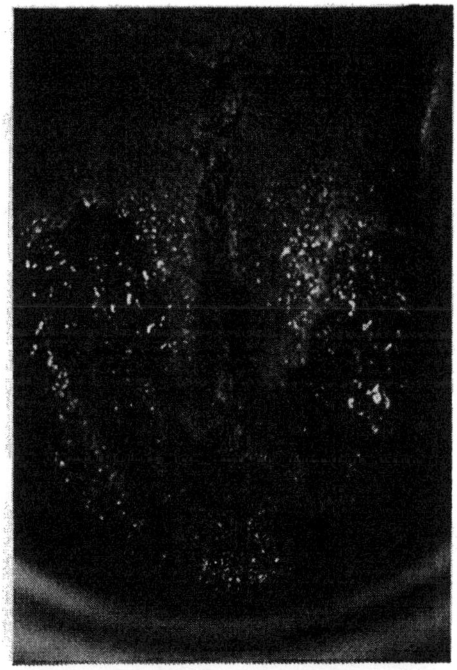

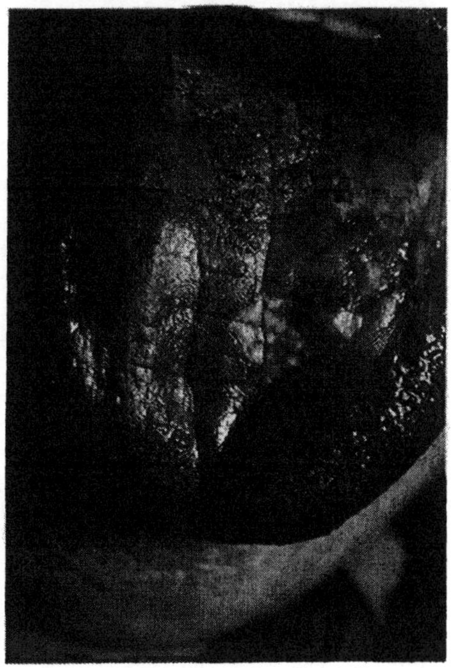

Colour photo 6. Erosive leukoplakia of the tongue in a 58-year-old female patient with glossitis associated with Plummer–Vinson syndrome which had been present for several years. This erosive lesion was identified histologically as carcinoma

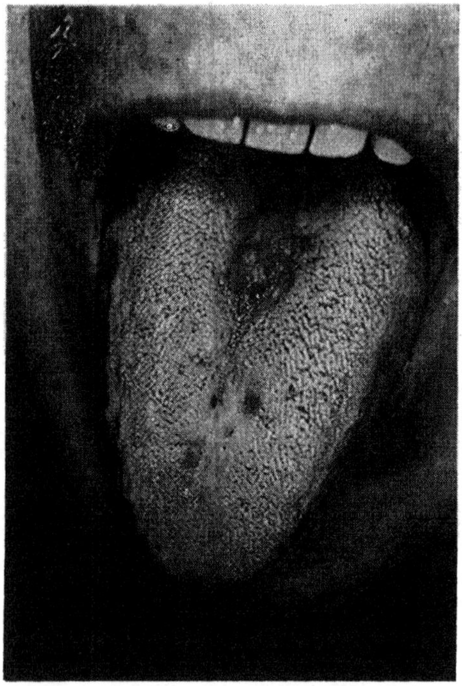

Colour photo 7. Median rhomboid glossitis in a 60-year-old male patient. The smooth, greyish-red, depapillated area on the dorsum of the tongue is healing after surgical excision of the lesion proper

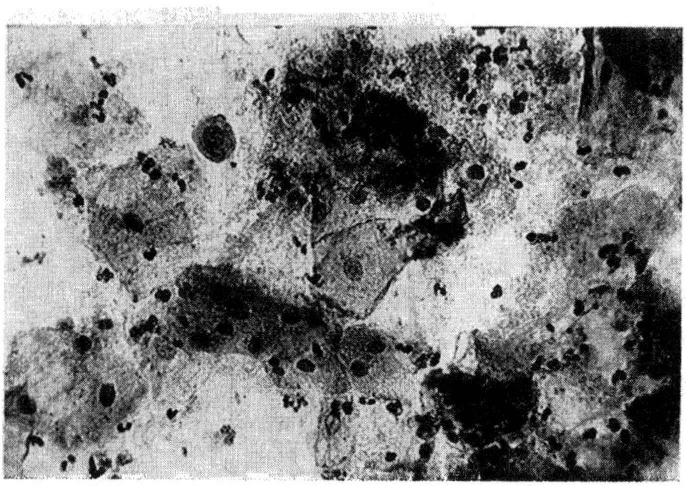

Colour photo 8. Cytological smear of scrapings from the lingual fissure seen in Fig. 40. Polymorphism, alteration of nuclear cytoplasmic ratio (→), and superficial parakeratosis (→). Papanicolaou's stain. ×340

Colour photo 9. Ulcer of the tongue in a 48-year-old male patient. The lesion developed in a leukoplakia which had been present for 20 years. The patient was a habitual smoker and an alcoholic

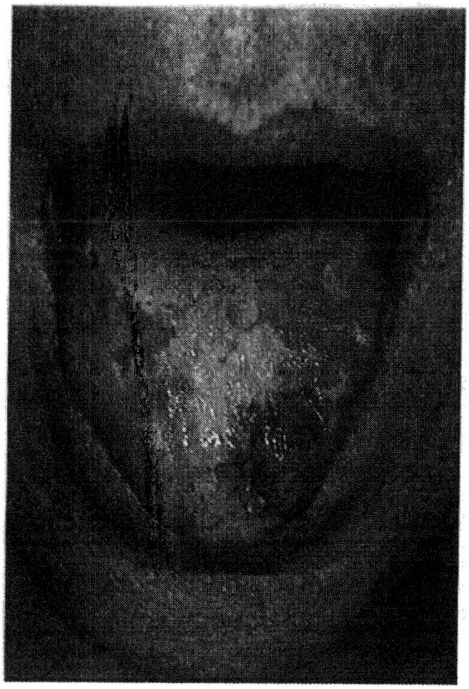

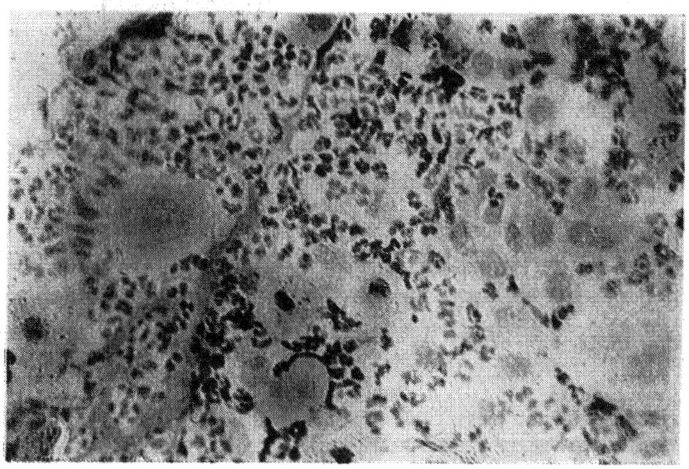

Colour photo 10. Cytological appearance of scrapings from the lingual ulcer shown on colour photo 9. Cellular polymorphism, anisocytosis, anisonucleosis, alteration of the nuclear : cyloplasmic ratio, orangeophilia. Papanicolaou's stain. $\times 340$

Colour photo 11. Reticular lichen in the buccal mucosa of a 64-year-old female patient. Note branching pattern of the papules

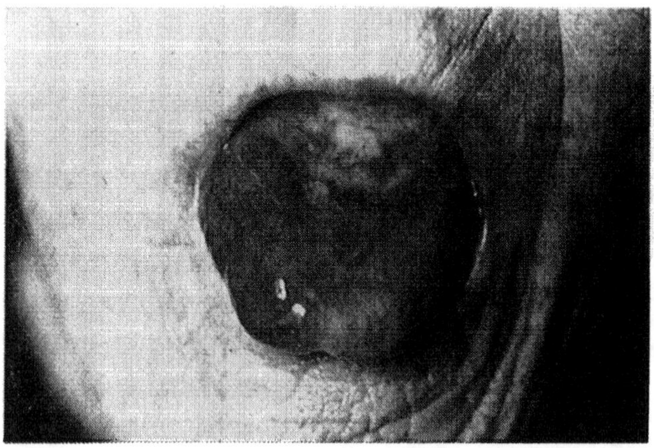

Colour photo 12. Atrophic lichen on the tongue of a 72--year-old female patient. The lesion had been present for several decades

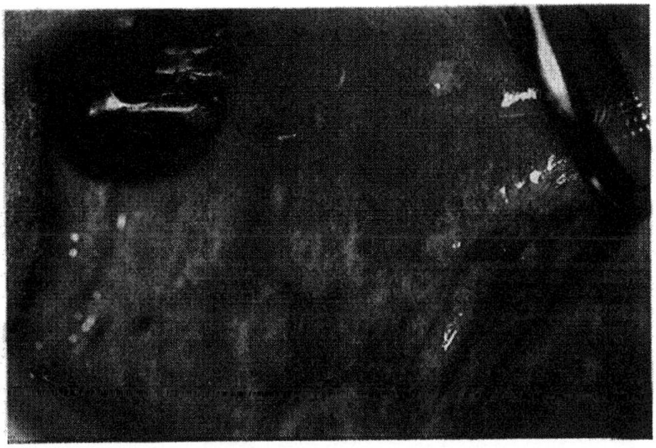

Colour photo 13. Erosive lichen in the buccal mucosa of a 45-year-old male patient

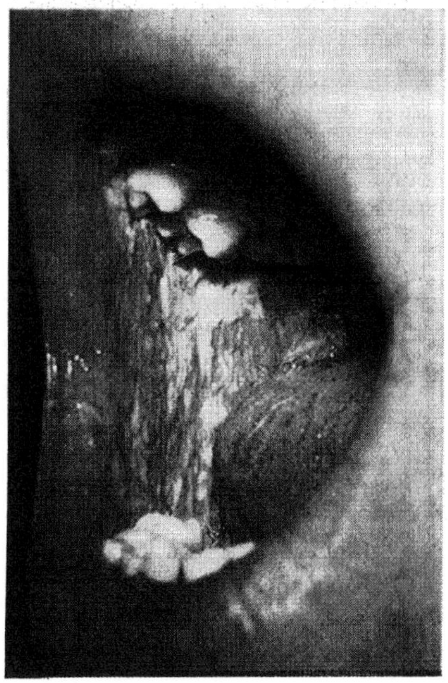

Colour photo 14. Leukoedema exfoliativum mucosae oris of a 23-year-old male patient. A soft white lesion with desquamating patches

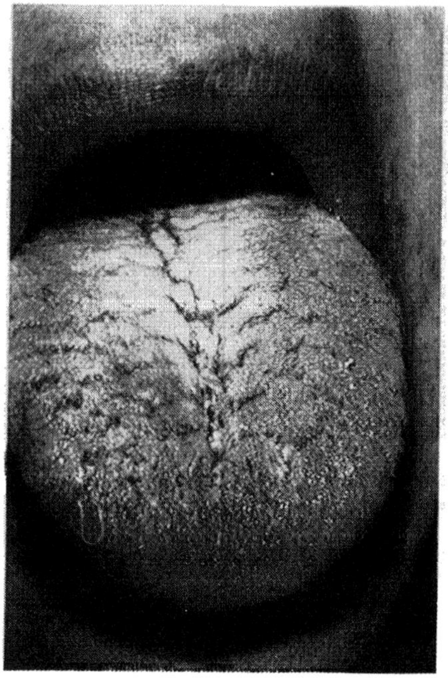

Colour photo 15. White sponge naevus on the dorsum of the tongue. The filiform papillae are elongated and keratinized, the fungiform papillae are prominent and swollen

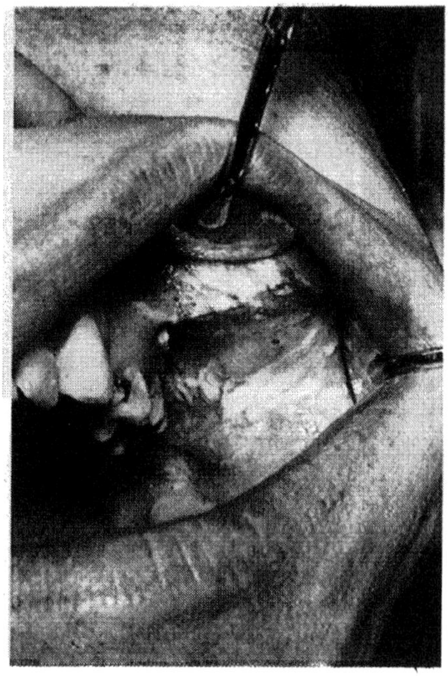

Colour photo 16. White sponge naevus in the vestibule (same patient as on colour photo 14)

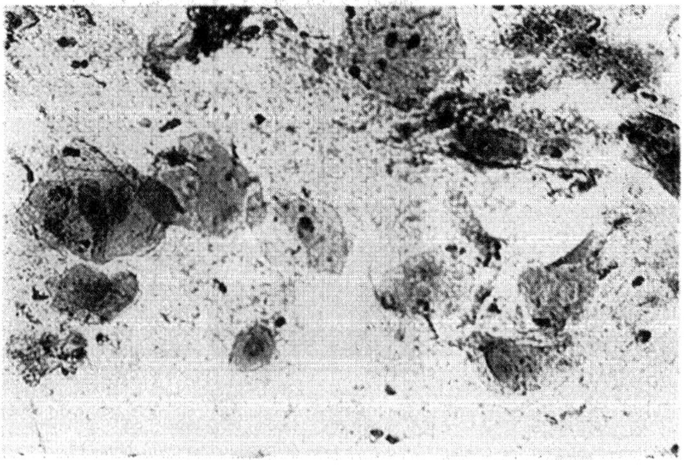

Colour photo 17. Cytological appearance of a smear from a buccal white sponge naevus. The cells are pale-staining and parakeratotic. Papanicolaou's stain. ×340

SUBJECT INDEX

GPSR Compliance
The European Union's (EU) General Product Safety Regulation (GPSR) is a set of rules that requires consumer products to be safe and our obligations to ensure this.

If you have any concerns about our products, you can contact us on

ProductSafety@springernature.com

In case Publisher is established outside the EU, the EU authorized representative is:

Springer Nature Customer Service Center GmbH
Europaplatz 3
69115 Heidelberg, Germany

www.ingramcontent.com/pod-product-compliance
Ingram Content Group UK Ltd.
Pitfield, Milton Keynes, MK11 3LW, UK
UKHW020954220926
475831UK00001B/71

* 9 7 8 9 4 0 0 9 7 5 6 6 8 *